GOD
CURES

GOD CURES

DAMON DAVIS

SILOAM

Most CHARISMA HOUSE BOOK GROUP products are available at special quantity discounts for bulk purchase for sales promotions, premiums, fund-raising, and educational needs. For details, write Charisma House Book Group, 600 Rinehart Road, Lake Mary, Florida 32746, or telephone (407) 333-0600.

GOD CURES by Damon Davis
Published by Siloam
Charisma Media/Charisma House Book Group
600 Rinehart Road
Lake Mary, Florida 32746
www.charismahouse.com

18 19 20 21 22 — 987654321
Printed in the United States of America

CONTENTS

ACKNOWLEDGMENTS

I HAVE SO MANY people to thank for their immense contribution to this journey. My ability to share this work with you is only made possible by my having successfully reached the other side of my own twenty-one-day journey.

It would only be fitting to begin with giving very special thanks to our God, the One who cures. Man's inability to treat an incurable autoimmune disease was overcome by God's miraculous healing power through the breakthrough strategies found in this book and as revealed to me by, from, and through so many powerful, intellectual, inspiring, and anointed leaders of our day.

I dedicate this work to some very special influences in my life: to my biological father, Wallace Ray Davis, who taught me how to fight and from whom I learned a "never say die" philosophy in the challenge to face life head on and courageously, staring fear, opposition, and negativity in the eyes; to my spiritual father, Creflo A. Dollar, a great and mighty general in God's kingdom, who stood in the gap for my legacy, taught me how my faith has the power to move mountains, and encouraged me to do what God has called me to do, to press in toward the never-ending, never-changing love and grace of a mighty God, and to not succumb to the enemy's prognosis for my future; to my grandfather, Bryan Webber, who taught me practical living and application of God's wisdom to every aspect of my life; and to my praying grandmother, Wedis, who taught me how to pray and to rest in the secret place and who is rallying for me in the heavenly places.

Pastor Gregory Dickow is someone very special who taught me that I have the power to change anything. He taught me that change comes from the inside out. He is a covenant friend and was my pastor for many years, and he taught me how to win the battle in my mind and that through conquering, I would find my calling.

My mother is the one who kept my dream alive for this work, my big encourager, the prognosticator of hope and possibility. She helped me in the struggle through the pain, fed me my medicine, helped me make my appointments, and kept reminding me along the way the real reason God was enabling me to walk this path.

Dr. Derek Grier is a great teacher of God's Word and has been my accountability leader along the way. His insight, mentorship, and transparency led me discover that a man can work himself silly trying to fix himself, when in fact only God is able, as the great Healer, to reach in deep and fix man once and for all.

Pastor Otoniel Font is the man God used to call out my destiny. He is my friend, my colleague, and my spiritual brother.

Special thanks to Pastor Frank Santora, whose prayers, wisdom, and encouragement contributed to my commitment to write *God Cures*. He is the man who told me it's never too late to do what God has called you to.

My good friend and fellow soldier Michael Orion Carter has been behind me in support of Legacy from the beginning. In an anointed manner, he helped me understand the importance of healing and how to receive it from the Lord.

My wife, Nathalie, was my rock in this storm—the one who told me that I could win, helped carry my chains, and sacrificed so much to help me discover me. My five children, whom I love so much, gave me the "what" it's all worth fighting for.

My brother, and my father's firstborn, Shannon Ray Davis, is a general on the battlefield of spiritual warfare! Charlie Campbell and M. Sean Anderson are my friends, business partners, late-night readers, commentators, and believers in this mission.

Special thanks to Don Roberts, a.k.a. Superman, the man God used mightily in the birth of Legacy Worldwide and who stood with me on the battlefield of Satan's attempt to kill it. My dear friend Jim Brown kept Psalm 91 before me and prayed it over me time after time. Scott Ulrich, Karen Brooks, Jenna Williams, and Jimmy Locklear were great contributors of ideas and sound bites that made it into my mind and into the pages of this work. A special shout out to Robert Downey Jr. for bringing my super-hero role model Iron Man to life!

Thanks to Kimberly Overcast and the team at Charisma Media. Special thanks to Steve Strang; without his belief in my vision to help the world discover how God can cure, you wouldn't be reading this.

Dr. Joseph Christiano, K. C. Craichy, Dr. Joe Clarino, Dr. Brian Wilmovsky, Dr. Caroline Leaf, and Dr. Joel Wallach came along-side me and surrounded me with the knowledge that transforms.

And finally, Dr. Daniel S. Stein left an impression that time cannot erase with his passionate pursuit to help humanity find the secret to looking good, living great, and loving well.

FOREWORD

IMAGINE LIVING IN a world where one exists in a constant state of emotional stagnation and dismay as well as the unawareness of one's disconnect of triune wholeness—physical, mental, and spiritual balance. But then by being more assertive and deliberate after thorough self-examination, self-awareness, and self-assessment, one can climb out of that emotional state by ultimately identifying and accepting one's immediate broken condition. And then with divine intervention, having strength and power with relentless tenacity, one can reach the pinnacle of emotional freedom by setting one's sights on something much higher than their circumstance—a cure.

Or imagine, in that same world, discovering how one can go from being ridden with pain, grossly incapacitated both physically and emotionally, into experiencing the utopia of physical and mental freedom that a pain-free life delivers, or furthermore experiencing how one can successfully turn desperation and daunting hopes of one day being in harmony and balance as the Creator intended by discovering a cure for whatever ails one's body, mind, and spirit!

Imagine living in that world where one can be taken from spiritual darkness and loneliness into a deeper and more intimate relationship with God, the Creator—a relationship that goes beyond Creator-creation and becomes a special relationship that meets the basic need for being and feeling loved, valued, and worthy, a father-child relationship.

Well, that is the world my longtime good friend and patient Damon Davis lived in and has transparently and exhaustively revealed in his book, *God Cures*.

As a naturopathic physician and seasoned veteran professional in natural health and wellness for nearly fifty years, I can personally as well as professionally attest to the frustrations, overwhelming roadblocks, and lack of answers to the myriad of questions that bog the minds of people from all walks of life who are in search of a cure—not some method of treating symptoms.

Conventional medical approaches to disease and degenerative illnesses (e.g., rheumatoid arthritis, multiple sclerosis, diabetes, and kidney failure) have had their place in treating humankind for decades and decades but reached their bell curve a long time ago. If one does not seek additional methods or approaches for healing, detoxification, regeneration, cellular repair, rejuvenation, etc., this conventional approach will only continue to cripple the mind of the person desperately seeking a remedy, a protocol to follow, or some way outside of the conventional box of thinking, and leave them in mental and physical despair. Unless the person with health issues and concerns has additional options and/or technologies available that can provide a better and more efficacious approach to their physical condition beyond treating symptoms, the probability of finding that cure is greatly reduced.

More than popping a pill or running a marathon or hitting the weights, a broader approach, perhaps even something that is "disruptive" in technology or innovation, is what smart patients will need to find the answers to their health-related dilemmas.

Our God and Creator made zero mistakes with His human creation. Humankind has been given all the genetic variableness to survive since Adam and Eve. And though man is gradually degenerating physically due to a litany of reasons, from environmental toxins to a multiplicity of diseases and illnesses to mental illness, etc., man intuitively and instinctively has found ways to combat this. Today we live in exciting times because of the cutting-edge technologies and therapies that are available to us (e.g., stem cell therapy and activation). There are many advanced nutritional and dietary protocols for one to take advantage of, exercise regimes for all types, dietary supplements, and much more that man has provided for procuring good health and vibrant living.

Combining the spiritual with the natural has always been a challenge for most people, particularly when it comes to one's health and physical condition. Is the only way for one to be healed found by going to the altar for healing? What about being a faithful caretaker of one's body as a form of worship, where the focus shifts from ourselves to Him?

What is clear to me in Damon's world and his book *God Cures* is that one's outcome in life is a combination of our heavenly Father's intervention and our willingness to be faithful with the clay He has given each of us. Our God and Creator uses His earthly human creation as instruments for healing and enhancing the physical and mental life of each one of us. But it is His supernatural love and power that brings about the ultimate remedy to what ails us in spirit, soul, and body. God cures!

—Dr. Joe Christiano, ND, CNC, CNHP

PREFACE

MY NAME IS Damon. I'm a fortysomething Caucasian, professional male, and prior to penning this book I was sick, diseased, and headed to an early grave, meaning death by the age of fifty. If your heart flatlining constitutes experiencing what death feels like, then I had that experience ten times before the age of twenty-five.

Dying, or the feeling of it, can really do something to your head. I lived past the age of twenty-five, but for reasons you will discover in this book I was essentially walking dead up until this journey. Despite battling sickness and disease since I was twenty-five, I am today in total recovery. I survived a heart issue in my twenties, but I was then diagnosed with an autoimmune disease that zapped me of energy, vitality, and emotional fortitude during critical years of my life. Nevertheless, today I am walking out the process of being cured, a term you will come to really understand in this book. Thanks to the chief architect, chemist, biologist, physicist, mathematician, artist, orchestrator, and Creator of it all, today I am thriving and able to help you thrive too.

I wrote this book for you, and I wrote it for two reasons, because of two words, *lonely* and *limited*, both of which I have learned to utterly despise. That means I have great contempt, or more eloquently, a deep repugnance for those two words, which describe the two feelings most likely swimming around you and which you, like I did at the beginning of my journey, have allowed to become your traveling partners in this thing called life. However, I refuse to leave you where I was; I refuse to leave you to the devices of these spirits of destruction. At the moment I realized how I became sick and by God's grace discovered a way out, I decided to tie a rope around the waist of as many people as possible to pull them out with me. When you picked up this book, you put a big rope around your waist. I'm going to pull it tight and pull you up before you put down this book.

Having walked an extraordinary path, I believe God has imparted to me an extraordinary revelation that will turn your life upside down and inside out for the better. I have written about my journey, demonstrating what it means when God cures and proving that He can cure you in twenty-one days too.

I wrote this book because of those two words that describe two realities, both of which we are going to destroy so you can live and abound as you never thought possible. The bedside companions *lonely* and *limited* must go. I've eradicated them from my own life, and I'm going to help you do the same as you embark upon this journey for yourself. No medication, no surgery, no therapist, and no theologian will be capable of giving you what only God can give. Like Elvis on a hot Vegas night, lonely and limited are leaving the building. We're pushing them out, never to return. Quite simply, God cures.

Being sick can be the loneliest place in the world. I mean *lonely*. Desert flower lonely. I never really understood how true this was, how lonely a world it is for the one who is sick, until I experienced my own health challenge.

You see, when we get sick, it's as though no one else is there with us. Sure, there may be lots of people around—family and friends—but when we are sick, it can feel as though we are utterly alone. The people closest to us at home, at work, and at church care about us with a certain level of sympathy; they show feelings toward us about our illness. But here's the deal: they lack true empathy. Sympathy is the same as pity, or better, it is compassion for what we, the sick, are walking through. Empathy is the ability to truly understand what it is that you and I are walking through.

Now, time out for a second, and then I'll return to my point. Acknowledging that sickness has befallen us is not an admission of defeat. For us faith-walkers, it is not ownership of it. I rebuke the devourer, and therefore I refuse to take hold or give title to whatever it is temporarily plaguing us. This journey is more about how to get out of where we are by taking ownership of how we got there. If we do not take ownership, we will end up right back where we were.

So, back to one being the loneliest number.

God is always ever present, just as David declared in Psalm 46:1: "God is our refuge and strength, a very present help in trouble." But in the natural sense, when you are sick, it can feel as though you are out on a raft in the great ocean of life with only your misery and pain to keep you company. It feels as if nowhere else in the world is lonelier. No one can really feel your pain. Your parents, your kids, your companion, your doctor, or your pastor can feel for you, but they don't feel what *you* feel. No one has to process the struggle mentally or emotionally like you do. No one is taking that insulin shot with you; no one is climbing the stairs with you and pushing through the pain. You go it alone. No one is in your head or feeling what is in your heart when you look at the world and watch others do what you cannot because you are in the prison of your own body.

But this loneliness goes deeper. The real *lonely* I am talking about is that there is not anyone who is going to focus on you like you will focus on you. To get well, it's going to take *you* to get you well. There are many people out there with a plan, a pill, or a program or who will drive you to the doctor's office and wait for you in the waiting room. But no one can do what it takes to get well for you. It's tough. It's difficult. It's a strenuous and emotional struggle to get over sickness, survive disease, and navigate yourself away from the fate Satan would have befall you. This process means that not only do you have to derail your plans for the present, in some cases putting your future on hold to do what has to be done to get well, but you will also have to push past the pain to lift your head every single day.

When you are sick, the closest people around you experience several stages of concern. They start out slowly. Unless you receive a major diagnosis, as in all of a sudden you definitely have this or that, then it may start with you lamenting about your symptoms, and they process it slowly. As the symptoms grow, they may start taking notice, and those closest to you will begin to care on a deeper level; this is when the sympathy kicks in. But soon enough the sympathy turns into something else. It was real for me, and it is real for you. When you are sick, feelings of sympathy can turn into feelings of annoyance, and you suddenly begin to feel like a burden. You may feel as though your illness is the albatross that hangs around the neck of your family and friends, and loneliness looms. These feelings of loneliness are real.

And then there's the other *L* word that deserves confrontation:

limited. This word sets the stage for a grand delusion, a master plan and diabolical plot of hell that I will explain fully and completely in the following pages. *Limited* means "confined" or "restricted."[1] It is when you are being held back and prevented from moving forward or progressing by some power. When sickness overcomes you, its grip, its pain, and its distraction limit you and hold you back.

Feeling lonely and limited is something that anyone and everyone at any level of affliction can understand, whether it is your health, your finances, or your relationships that are ailing, or if you simply lack the courage and confidence to do what your heart tells you to do. I wrote this book to help you overcome the loneliness and limitation you have experienced when your spirit, soul, or body is attacked.

I fought loneliness and limitation valiantly. I met them on the battlefield, I stared them right in the eyes, and I defeated them once and for all. And I want this victory for you. You see, it was not the physical manifestation of my sickness that compelled me to find a cure; it was the stark revelation of how strong loneliness and limitation had become in my life, and having discovered how to defeat them, I simply cannot and will not leave anyone where I once was.

Across the water at Hickam Air Force Base on the beautiful island of Oahu in Hawaii, there is a military agency called the Defense POW/MIA Accounting Agency (DPAA). Each and every year the DPAA spends millions of dollars not for search-and-rescue missions but to find and collect the remains of soldiers who died in wars that have long since been over.[2] I celebrate what we do for those who died in the service of our country, but it is the deeply rooted, unrelenting proposition of "leave no man behind" that really jumps out at me about what this military agency does. It is this kind of commitment that really gives me pause.

In practicing the principle of leaving no one behind, I must first focus on those who are alive and still on the battlefield, fighting every day and struggling to find some semblance of hope to keep fighting another day. Perhaps that is you.

Ecclesiastes 9:4 captures it well. While there is breath, there is hope. Hope is sometimes all there is for us to hold on to.

It's time to fight. The fact that God can cure is real. That's your hope. And hope is closely tied to faith. Hebrews 11:1 tells us, "Now faith is the substance of things hoped for, the evidence of things not seen." Together we are going to fight with hope and faith, knowing that God has got your back. He has heard your prayers, and He has a plan for your complete and total restoration.

God has set you up for the greatest days of your life. Whether you realize it or not, sickness is part of the enemy's strategy to limit you, to prevent you from fulfilling the purposes of God for your life. I discovered the truth of that statement, and I determined that I was not going to allow the enemy to prevent me from becoming the leader God created me to be or stop me from discovering the God-created purpose written on the tablets of my heart.

I wrote this book to carve a path that you can follow. The rope is around your waist. Now help me—hang on as I pull you. Your future awaits. Success leaves clues. Let's follow the path that Jesus walked, following His footsteps into the victory He has prepared for you.

INTRODUCTION

S O, WHERE DID it all begin? Healing began the day I declared, "I am healed." Nevertheless, it was not until I tapped into the revelation profiled in this book that I became free of disease, cured by God in twenty-one days.

"I am healed." There is power in your words, and this declaration is one of dominion. God gave you the authority to declare a thing as so, and it is so! Hebrews 2:8 says, "'You have put all things in subjection under his feet.' For in subjecting all things under him, He left nothing that is not subjected to him" (MEV). And Psalm 8:6 says, "You have given him dominion over the works of Your hands; You have put all things under his feet" (MEV).

We are not looking for a treatment. We are not looking for remission. We are looking for a total eradication of the disease that plagues your body. Through a twenty-one-day journey, God is going to show you how you will be cured and stay that way—completely free from sickness and disease for the rest of your days.

Allow me to begin by making some things clear before you dive into chapter 1. First, this is not another strict diet program that you cannot stick to. I am drinking a double shot latte with one sugar as I write, and last night I wolfed down a hamburger. Yes, you can relax. This book is about balance. I just have a lot fewer hamburgers than I once did. I discovered a lot about food and the quote about it attributed to Hippocrates: "Let food be thy medicine and medicine be thy food."[1] Said my way, "Food kills, and food heals." God's supernatural download into my spirit about this truth is truly what has cured me. However, as it pertains to diet (what to eat and what not to eat), let me state clearly and for the record that if God, who knows everything about our bodies and how they work, expected us to live on fruits and nuts and veggies alone, then He would not have had Jesus feed a multitude with bread and fish. (See Matthew 14:13–21.)

While there are certainly some very clear things to try to avoid pertaining to diet, exercise, prayer, meditation, and exploring and discovering happiness through hobbies and joy through Jesus, this book is more about things we can do to improve our condition without becoming religious about it and completely restricting all the little things that give us pleasure in life. Throughout this process I discovered some good old-fashioned common sense from Scripture. I also learned from the experience and expertise of many of the greatest minds and from the mentors in my life, including Creflo Dollar (my spiritual father), Pastor Gregory Dickow, Cindy Trimm, Sam Chand, Derek Grier, A. R. Bernard, Pastor Michael Freeman, Pastor Frank Santora, Pastor Otoniel Font, Bill Winston, Apostle Renny McLean, Pastor Benny Hinn, Evangelist Daniel Kolenda, Pastor Jentezen Franklin, Dean Graziosi, Brad Richdale, Les Brown, Mother

Teresa, Billy Graham, Bishop Keith Butler, Pastor Tony Brazelton, David Jeremiah, Rick Warren, and many others.

I discovered a life of happiness through balance, through God's grace but not religion. I like what A. R. Bernard says about what happiness really is: "Happiness isn't a commodity that can be purchased in a store; it's a by-product of the way you choose to live and the things you choose to think." To put it simply, I like eating. But I believe that God made food for us to enjoy, so you're not going to go on the cardboard diet to get healthy. You're going to understand what food really is, what food is not, what living right and thinking right is, how to find what is right for your body, how to take care of your body, and how to get aligned in your triune man, along with discovering God's original intent with the wonderful and amazing creation He set before us to master and take dominion of until eternity comes.

Second, this is also a scientific book. It is full of expertise that you need to understand about how your body, the temple of the Holy Spirit, was made. I promise it will not be a snoozefest. If this book was solely opinion based, it would merely mirror many self-help books that just offer you the author's perspective. No, this book is based upon facts, evidence, and real science that experts across the globe agree are real and work. What you will learn here is revolutionary, and when the light goes off in your head by being exposed to the truth that the establishment (and Satan) wants to hide from you, you will want to share this with everyone you know.

Third, though I am not a doctor, I have been surrounded by them through the years of my journey to discover God's cure. This book is not intended to treat or cure any disease. This book is intended to prove that God's cure exists and is available to anyone who is hungry enough and ready enough to find it! I believe you will find your answers here. Don't stop taking your medicine (if the doctor tells you to keep taking it), and don't avoid seeing the doctor if you think you need to see one. If anything, this book will assist you in navigating conventional wisdom and better understanding conventional medicine while simultaneously exposing you to the truth that many medical professionals have yet to fully grasp. I call this *revelation*. As my colleague Joel Wallach says, "Dead doctors don't lie."[3]

And last but certainly not least, this book is about God. I am referring to the Christian one. If you are atheist, agnostic, or religion-specific and not of the Christian persuasion, I encourage you to look beyond your prejudices and give this book a chance. I ask you to explore the unknown with me. Why not? You have tried everything else, right? This won't hurt, I can assure you.

So, when did it all begin for you? It's important to try to remember when you noticed a difference, when things stopped being normal and you adapted to a new normal. You used to sleep through the night, you were able to eat anything you wanted without heartburn, you could run and leap, you laughed, you could move easily without pain, and you could bend down and tie your shoes without getting winded. You used to look forward to the future, and you used to dream big dreams. Remember?

We have all been living in the new and unimproved version of ourselves for so long that we cannot really remember much of how we used to look or how we used to feel. But your diagnosis and the medication you are on to keep functioning are not God's plan or will for your life. Your condition is not just part of aging. Your struggle with health, happiness, money, or relationships is not just life. It is completely possible for God to cure whatever you need cured.

My Story

I woke up one morning and couldn't move. When I say I couldn't move, I mean literally I couldn't move. I was on my six-thousand-dollar mattress, one of those memory foam jobs they price really high and sell easily because they promise you will have the best dreams of your life and wake up feeling refreshed, full of energy, and ready to take on the day. I was no stranger to products that promised they would change your world if you would only call now and place your order. And there I was, a customer who had purchased miracle-working memory foam. But that day the memory foam was not working miracles.

I woke up looking out the third-floor window of my Victorian home in downtown Jacksonville, Florida. The birds were chirping, and the sun was shining. But I just couldn't move. My hands were so tight they could not close to make a fist. My legs were so stiff (which I would later discover was from inflammation) that they would not bend. My neck was stiff, my back was stricken with pain, and my breathing was labored. Fear covered me like a heated blanket in the middle of winter, and for a moment I wondered if I was still dreaming. I was not dreaming. I was very much awake, and I couldn't move. I was terrified.

Thirty minutes passed while I was immobile and in pain, but no one was home. My wife had already taken the kids to school and gone on to work. I was by myself, and I wondered for a moment if these were my final hours. After another thirty minutes, I worked my legs off the bed and onto the floor. (I later found out my body's inflammation was finally dissipating.) I managed to push myself up and stand despite excruciating, sharp pain in my feet, as if I were standing on glass. I sat back down quickly with my feet dangling off the large bed with the expensive mattress that was supposed to cure all, and I wondered what was wrong. My eyes were watering profusely. I was hot. I seemed to have a fever. I knew that something was wrong.

I had just returned from a humanitarian endeavor—a trip to the Congo with Dikembe Mutombo, the seven-foot-two, world-renowned, Congolese-American NBA Hall of Famer with shoes so big you could fit a pair of my shoes inside each one. Dikembe arrived in this country and entered the basketball scene with passion. He achieved success nearly every single time his feet graced the court. When he retired, he focused his attention back on his homeland with a mission to help his people. In honor of his dear mother and with a heart to help the people of the Democratic Republic of Congo, he built a three-hundred-bed hospital in the capital, Kinshasa; the Biamba Marie Mutombo Hospital was the first modern medical facility built in Kinshasa in almost forty years.[4]

When the hospital celebrated its grand opening, I was invited to produce and host a documentary about this miraculous and much-celebrated occasion. It was a trip that I was proud to be part of. I walked through villages meeting the people of the Congo and discovering the war-torn country's conditions. It was a place where medicine was scarce, rations were low, and children struggled for survival. The things we consider in this country to be commonplace, like cream for your coffee, were an unheard-of luxury to these people. The beautiful, sweet people of the Congo suffered through the aftermath of many wars, diminished access to clean drinking water, and a minimal level of medical care available. Dikembe set out to help solve the medical care problem, and I hosted a nationally televised documentary to tell the world about it.

So as I lay in my bed, unable to move, I wondered if something in the Congo triggered the sickness that had befallen my body. I remembered one shot from the opening of the program where I had to step one hundred yards into the Congo River and wondered if something had gotten inside me from the water. I know you've seen the movies where this happens, and your imagination can run wild when you are sick. You start feeling pain somewhere, and before you know it, according to your Google search, you're dying.

Was it the twelve different vaccinations I had for my trip that had somehow ripped my body apart by dumping small traces of several diseases into my bloodstream? Diseases such as yellow fever, malaria, and polio have been eradicated in the United States, but they have remained alive and well in parts of Africa. At that moment, I had no idea what was wrong, but it was the start of my journey.

This story is my story. It is my story of getting sick, somewhere, somehow, sometime in my past. It is a story of my discovery of where it began and how I tunneled my way out, against the odds, to where I am today—living a life in which I am not just surviving but thriving. It is a journey you can follow. And listen to me: it can work every time and for anyone.

DISCOVERING THE CAUSE OF SICKNESS

My story actually does not begin in the Congo or even lying in a bed unable to move. My story begins much earlier than that, and together we will take a journey into the recesses of my past to find out the real cause of my sickness—a sickness that was life-threatening and potentially debilitating. And note this: the doctors called it incurable.

This is my journey of discovery to find out how we, humanity, become sick. And if you are reading this book, if you are sick and diseased, if you have ever been given a diagnosis with a death sentence, then I invite you to take this same life-changing journey. Together we will discover that God cures.

I know that you're tired and perhaps downtrodden, discouraged, and depressed. You're sick. And like so many—and like me at the outset of this journey—you may be overcome with fear. I know how you feel because I *was* you. I wrote this book to help you bring restoration to your body, restoration to your mind, healing to your heart, happiness to your soul, and joy to your spirit by bringing the three parts of your total composition, spirit, soul, and body, into perfect alignment. Let this journey lead you back to the way God created you, back to the ancient paths, back to a time and a place where the Creator's original intent and design for you can be fully restored. God can heal you.

So I invite you to learn about my story and how I overcame sickness by uncovering the truth of how our spirits, souls, and bodies should function and work together and how getting them into a state of proper alignment can move us directly into healing. We can move into a place that science, biology, and physics define as homeostasis, where we, the created ones, are engineered to heal ourselves. What you discover in this book will challenge your thinking. It will provoke new thought. It might, in fact, even fly in the face of and rival some conventional thought, exposing you to new ideas, all of which will align perfectly with God's Word. This book contains wisdom from many experts whom I have come to know, many of whom I call friends and who walked beside me on this journey that exposed me to revelation and truth that you may not be able to find simply by exploring the textbooks.

I have been on a journey of discovery for many years. I uncovered some mysteries that perhaps are being revealed to us in the fullness of God's time. And this book, with its information and revelation pulled from the four corners of the globe and gleaned from ancient manuscripts, will reveal to you the steps to take to overcome your illness, push back disease, and allow God to cure.

You and I were not created for sickness. We were not designed to die. That was not God's plan and intent. From the very foundations of time when God spoke you and me into existence, beginning with the man and woman in the garden, we were created to live for all eternity. And despite the fall of man in the garden, God's love and His plans for you have not changed—plans to live an abundant life, where you are happy, where you are healthy, where you are whole. The true definition of *prosperity* that my spiritual father, Creflo Dollar, reminds me of often is "nothing missing, nothing broken; everything whole."

As you read this book, you will discover that this type of living, this type of thinking, this type of doing, this kind of existence, this paradigm, is *possible*. Doctors will not explain it to you because they do not understand it. The gurus of New Age and new thought do not understand it, so they cannot explain it to you. A life coach or motivational speaker who speaks about what this world can offer you cannot explain it to you. But I have turned over every rock and sought the mentorship of the wise to help me grasp how and why we fall victim to disease so easily and how we can get out of it and live that life of prosperity the Bible declares and decrees is available to you.

In these pages you will be exposed to an insight that will change who you are. It will change the way you think, the way you act, the way you love, and the way you look. It will revitalize your soul and give you spiritual perspective as your spirit takes control, assumes its rightful place of governing your soul; your soul then, with the leading of the spirit, will govern your body. You will, day by day, be conformed to the image of your Creator, and your life will begin again. Your life will begin again. It's time for us to look good, live great, and love well.

For some, perhaps for you, these words seem foreign and unfamiliar. They are perhaps promises you have never heard before or never quite understood. It will be the beginning of a new life, a life that the Creator meant for you. There are no empty promises on these pages. Empty promises are made by people who never made the journey. I made the journey. I walked the Damascus Road. I have seen the traces of footsteps on the dirt path where Paul traveled from blindness into an ever-increasing light. My discovery is not new, but it is foundational and timeless. It is a promise from your Creator; it is His design and destiny for you.

If you allow it, this book will dive deep into the core of who you are and reveal what is standing in your way of reaching the true peace and joy God wants for you. It will become a tool, a blueprint, a guiding light to help you find your way in the dark of night through troubled waters and lead you to health, happiness, and prosperity. This will be one of the most painful, thought-provoking, and in-your-face steps you have ever taken, but it will prove to be the one of the most revealing and life-transforming journeys you have ever embarked upon. It will reveal to you how to transcend life by championing everything and anything that comes at you. It will lead you to the most incredible pinnacle of empowerment to conquer your future and live a courageous life.

In writing this book, I am hoping to help all of us connect with the Creator and bring our bodies, souls, and spirits into the unity, alignment, and balance He originally intended. As the doors open through understanding, as the truth about what this life is all about begins to transcend your circumstances, you will discover what I have. Although pain may be an inevitable part of this life, with the right mind and a pure heart, and with your spirit leading your soul and your soul governing your body, your pain, your story, your struggle, and your testimony of where you were and where you are will become the greatest advantage to help you lead others out of their own darkness and into the light.

To make it through this book, you have to allow its revelation to activate itself in your life. You must therefore check your cynicism at the door. You have to put your doubt on pause and release your grip on control. You must set in your mind that this is an important book, and you must commit to finish it.

Let's go.

Chapter 1

LOOKING FOR ANSWERS

I F ONLY WHEN we were born they could have embedded an information chip in our brains so all the answers to living the good life could have been accessible in milliseconds. Instead, we often have to wait. Such is the case with those of us working our way out and through to becoming healthy. My grandmother talked about having to cook on a wood-burning stove when she was a child. It took an hour to make a meal. With a microwave you can make a meal in a matter of minutes, but the meal certainly will not be as tasty. When I was six, I had to get off the couch and walk across the room to change the channel on Saturday morning during the cartoon stretch. Today we stay on the couch and push a button on a remote. And we can even eliminate the commercials if we watch on the Internet.

But getting answers on how to live and navigate life's tough spots, such as getting into college, financing a car, buying a house, doing your taxes, or making marriage work, usually means taking the long way around to get the answers you need. And in many cases, it's only experience that gives you the answers you need. It's hindsight. And hindsight is always twenty-twenty; your vision is not impaired. Imagine for a second how many things you would do differently, the decisions you would have made differently, if only you had that chip in your brain with all the answers. If I ever invent one, I will call it the twenty-twenty chip. It will be the chip that has the culmination of one hundred people's life experiences, all of whom have lived to tell the story of how to navigate the troubled waters of life. No more going into uncharted terrain. All you need is that twenty-twenty chip to live the victorious life!

But then again, thanks to technology, when you need something such as a phone number or even an answer to a tough question, you can just open up a search browser on your phone or laptop and get an answer. Whatever it is, just go to a search engine and type in the question, or whatever you need, and in seconds you've got an answer. Of course, you usually get more than you need. There might be hundreds of different options, answers, comments, or votes on a topic, and suddenly the options and answers are more confusing than your original question.

I saw a commercial about a talking box (that is what my grandfather would call it if he saw it). It basically has voice-detecting technology that allows you to ask whatever question you have, and it will answer the question for you audibly in seconds. This two-way intelligent speaker, when connected to the Internet, will do many things, but two specifically: First, it will play your music on command. Just tell it what song you want, and it will play it. Second, you can ask it do something, and it will perform the command, such as setting an alarm for a certain time or ordering household supplies. I am going to buy one. But what's my point?

Isn't God's Word supposed to be like the twenty-twenty chip? Isn't the Bible a compilation of a bunch of folks' lives and journeys and how God directed their lives and ordered their steps? And as such, is it not a road map for us? Doesn't the Bible give us perfect vision? Doesn't it give us the answers when we need them? Doesn't it tell us how to make it through the troubled waters of life and how to live victoriously?

WHEN YOU WANT ANSWERS

Sometimes there's a problem. It seems that accessing the information is not always easy, and for some reason when I need an answer to a problem right now, the processing speed seems to be really slow. I wish we had get-it-quick results when we need an answer from God. I wish that when we read the Word or prayed, the answer would come quickly and be extremely clear. "Do this. Don't do that."

I have a feeling you want that too. You may be expecting a sermon about waiting on God—He's always on time, and He's never late—but that is not where I'm headed. Because sometimes you want something different than a "just in time" God. If only on that dark morning when I woke to the symptoms of sickness raging in my body I could have talked to God like that talking box. I would have said, "Hey, God?" He would have replied, "Yes, My son?" It would have been audible; I could have heard Him with my ears. I would have asked, "So what's going on in my body? Tell me what to do so that it will go away." And God could have answered, "Sure, you are sick. It's in this place or that, and this is why. Here's what you need to do, and you will be better in two hours." If only that could have happened. Or even if I could have responded, "Hey, God? That's too much work. Just heal me now," and God could have said, "OK. You are healed."

But God is not a talking box. So instead, I anguished. I cried hard. All I could think was, "Will I ever catch a break? Will there always be suffering for me? What did I do to deserve this? Haven't I already gone through enough?"

Let's see…I survived a serious illness when I was four years old. I survived my parents' divorce, which was violent and devastating. I survived child abuse by a drunken stepfather who beat me daily with a belt buckle in the boiler room of our house. I survived moving two times every year while I was school-age. I survived heart disease in my early adulthood that led to my heart stopping twelve times before the age of twenty-seven. I could go on.

So I cried out to God for minutes that turned to hours that turned to days that turned to weeks, months, and years. If only God would have answered like voice-detecting technology. But life, it seems, is never that easy. God is there. We know this with the certainty found in Matthew 28:20, where it tells us that He is with us always. But in truth, when we are sick and need answers, it does not always feel as though God is an ever-present help in times of trouble, as the Word promises in Psalm 46:1.

None of us want to be limited and in pain, and I don't want to wait until the end of days to be free from the chains of sickness or disease. Revelation 21:4 says that God will personally "wipe away every tear from their eyes, and death shall be no more, neither shall there be mourning, nor crying, nor pain anymore, for the former things have passed away" (ESV).

And the truth is that *God is there.* He is sitting at your bedside. He is fully and completely aware that you are struggling, and although He might not respond like the talking box, God always responds to you. Be encouraged that God is there with you now. He has your back. He loves you with an unconditional love, and no matter how bleak things might seem, believe me when I tell you that your best days are ahead of you. But why the wait? Perhaps He wants to teach us something. Perhaps He wants to cure us, not just heal us. *Heal. Cure.* What's the difference?

Going Deeper

I believe the answers for my situation were there with God all along, and He was waiting on me to really press in. God had the answers, and He was waiting on me to access them. To teach me what I needed to know, He needed me to go deeper. I believe God wanted to show me something. God needed to teach me something. But technology like the talking box has removed the need to make a real effort to get the answers to life's questions. Instead, with minimal effort we get what we need. Yet so often we get what we need for the moment, but we miss getting what we need for a lifetime.

Did you get that? God does not want to give us just a simple solution for right now. He wants to teach us how to see differently and how to process differently, and through those means to create with Him and through Him a life that is abundant, that is lived fully and lived until eternity. If God were only working with us to focus on what we need now, and if He were only to rescue us in the midst of the trial, we would learn nothing. It is kind of like the stories of people who win the lottery. They are broke, but then they scratch and win millions of dollars. After a year or two, they are broke again. What happened? Well, sometimes in order to learn, we have to *earn* it. If we learn it because we earned it, we appreciate it. If we appreciate it, we respect it. If we respect it, we protect it. If we protect it, it has a tendency to last. And if it lasts, we are able to pass it along.

But since technology has made it so that we do not have to wait anymore, we have forgotten that sometimes God wants to stop us, slow us down, and get us to think more deeply about what is really going on in our lives because He wants to give us the answer that gets to the root of our problems and fixes them once and for all.

When we do not look deeper beneath the surface, when we do not rethink things and consider that things are wrong because what we have been taught is wrong, we keep making the same mistakes and passing the same issues from one generation to the next. I like how Oswald Chambers said it: "It is not true to say that God wants to teach us something in our trials. Through every cloud He brings our way, He wants us to *unlearn* something."[1] Wow. That's a better answer than the talking box could ever give us! When we give God our all, when we press in to Him, when we surrender, He gives us something that changes us.

> For those whom he foreknew he also predestined to be con-
> formed to the image of his Son, in order that he might be
> the firstborn among many brothers.
> —ROMANS 8:29, ESV

I love the story about Peter stepping out of the boat when Jesus called to him. I have heard it preached so many times and in so many ways. Many point out that Peter needed to keep his eyes on Jesus. And then there is the point that Peter had to get out of the boat to walk on water; that one also gets a lot of notice. And both points are solid and true.

My view is certainly not new, but it is how I see Peter's story in context of what I am trying to show you. Peter learned that it was imperative to keep his eyes on Jesus. This one is straightforward, and we all get it. But why was it imperative? Beyond the obvious reason, why was it important to keep his eyes on Jesus? I believe Jesus wanted Peter to understand that his answers could only come from the Master.

This one is spot on. While sometimes our answers may come indirectly from Him, nonetheless all good things that are for our benefit come from Jesus. If man is empowered or receives a revelation, it is still from God.

> Every good and perfect gift is from above, coming down from the Father of the heavenly lights, who does not change like shifting shadows.
>
> —JAMES 1:17, NIV

So if we know where our answer is coming from, then why do we try to rush God? I believe there are generally two reasons. First, we are in a lot of pain and do not want to wait on Jesus. Second, we think we already have the answer and therefore don't need Him. That last one really gets us messed up. We often take the route that most people are talking about, the one that gets us to the answer the quickest, with less struggle, less pain, and less cost.

But that is nothing short of second-guessing God. And many people who are sick end up playing this second-guessing game or else playing the waiting game with the medical establishment long before they ever get to the real answer of what is wrong. We are going to get to the root of that in this book.

THE CYCLE OF ILLNESS

I am not suggesting that we avoid the route of conventional medicine. In fact, I often think we need to move faster to engage our doctor or an expert before things get worse. The issue we are going to deal with in this book, however, is that we typically find ourselves treating the symptoms of illness without ever really

7

getting to the root of what caused our sickness to begin with. Getting a quick answer rather than the right answer and the complete answer leads to a cycle of illness. We treat the symptoms and medicate the pain, often creating new problems while failing to address the root issue. It is a vicious, never-ending cycle. And because billions of dollars are at stake, the medical and pharmaceutical industries would nearly be out of business if we actually got well and stayed well.

Meanwhile, we are caught in a cycle that goes something like this:

1. Experience symptoms.

2. Make an appointment with the doctor.

3. Go to the doctor's office, fill out paperwork, pay co-pay, get vitals checked and blood drawn, wait for results, and receive no diagnosis.

4. Get referred to a specialist, fill out more paperwork, pay another co-pay, get more blood drawn, and perhaps have some tests run. Wait for results.

5. Return to the doctor, pay another co-pay, receive no real diagnosis, get a prescription for some medicine to try, and schedule next appointment.

6. Go to the pharmacy, pay co-pay, and get medicine.

7. Repeat step 5.

8. Repeat step 6.

Is anyone tired of this cycle? Does anyone find the whole thing confusing and frustrating?

I believe God was teaching me to understand what sickness and disease are at a cellular level. I am fully convinced that my thorn in the flesh was necessary. The answers were found with God. Yes, I was speaking to Him, but I was expecting Him to talk to me the way I wanted Him to talk to me. I was expecting Him to take my problem away. God wanted me to unlearn some things, and He wanted to reveal something new to me. God wanted to show me something that would shift everything in my life, and He did.

God wanted me to discover what sickness really was, what healing was, and how He wanted to cure me.

ON THE ROAD TO DAMASCUS

I woke one morning after returning from another international trip. I was very swollen, and my joints, especially in my hips and my legs, were so tight I could barely move. I managed to put my feet on the floor after a while, but it felt like I was stepping on razor blades. I maneuvered back into a lying position with my head on my pillow and waited awhile, moving slowly but more and more over the course of an hour, allowing the inflammation in my body to subside. This whole episode scared me nearly to death. I still wonder to this day why I didn't call 911. It was probably for the same reason we procrastinate when symptoms arise, telling us that something is wrong in the body: we hope that whatever it is will just go away. Fear and stubbornness is not a good combination.

So there I was, temporarily disabled. Over the next few days it happened again. I went to see a rheumatologist, who took blood work and after a few weeks gave me a diagnosis that really did not make me happy: "I have no idea what's wrong with you."

The closest I got to an actual diagnosis was that I had an autoimmune disease. One doctor was fully convinced by all my symptoms that I had rheumatoid arthritis. He put me on highly toxic immunosuppressant medication, basically to turn off my immune system because it was attacking my body. I found it strange that my father had been on similar medication following his heart transplant.

I spent years on a road to Damascus, waiting on God, pleading with Him, but my approach was all wrong. I wanted God to answer me like the talking box. I wanted Him just to fix me—but I was not interested in getting to the root and dealing with the core issues that set everything in motion.

So what were my core issues? Essentially I was a broken-down mess.

I was a workaholic and made very little room for God. I did not pray regularly. I was not reading my Bible. I had little time for church. I was hot-tempered and intolerant, and I had an insatiable need for everything to be perfect—even though I wasn't. I was never satisfied; nothing was ever good enough.

I ate too much, and I ate the wrong stuff. (It does not take a degree in nutrition to know some of the really bad stuff for our bodies. Everyone knows that a triple cheeseburger with large fries and a Coke is bad for you.) I never worked out; I absolutely despised it. My exercise consisted of walking in the airport between flights. I never got any sun. I'm a cave dweller. If there isn't air-conditioning, I'll pass.

I was not a good husband, although I told myself I was. I took care of my family's financial needs, which seemed to be my only job, but in chasing that, I lost sight of everything else. If I am completely honest with myself, which is an important part of getting cured, I have to admit that I was a lame father.

There is more, but you get the picture. So, there I was, writhing in pain. My body was inflamed. My body temperature was often as high as one hundred and one degrees. My back hurt always. My knees hurt. My feet hurt. My hands hurt. Even my tailbone hurt. I woke every day to the same pain, immobility, limitation, and frustration.

I was waiting on God to fix me, but what I really wanted God to do was just make my sickness go away. I was waiting passively and without responsibility. You see, we cannot simply hope something good will happen and just sit there until it does. Sometimes God expects us to be active in getting our answers. There are times when we indeed just rest in the arms of the Almighty and wait while the God of great grace and mercy does what He does behind the scenes, but there are times we have to do something. We have to cooperate with the Master. This is not about works, and I am not disputing the fact that grace is at work always and we have God's unmerited favor. I am speaking to a responsibility we have to be responsible for ourselves. I was not looking to fix myself; I was looking for God to simply fix my problem. But there are times we have to look deeper, go deeper, and do deeper than before, especially when we are sick. Yes, faith works, but as James 2:26 tells us, "Faith without works is dead."

But I believe there was something else God was doing in me and for me. He was trying to show me something by doing something in me. Much as Paul saw that his sufferings revealed Christ's power was made perfect in his weakness, I believe God was trying to get me to rely on His strength to get me through. Why? Because if and when I could see that it was God who cured me, I would know that only God could have cured me. As a result, I would know that what I endured had a purpose—to enable me to reveal that God cures to other sick people who face the same struggles that I did.

God struck me down in the middle of the road, blinded me to what man said was my problem, and opened my eyes to the answer: Him. I cannot count the number of times I sat in a waiting room or how much money I spent on pills. It is sad to say, but one of the compelling reasons I stopped taking my last round of medication and decided to break down was that the toxicity of what they prescribed was causing immense intestinal and digestive issues in my body, and my hair was falling out. Let me tell you, that last one will do the trick any day of the week.

AT THE ALTAR

So one day I boarded a plane and flew to Chicago, Illinois, to see a man in whom I had tremendous confidence spiritually. His name is Pastor Gregory Dickow. Pastor Dickow was not only a spiritual leader in my life, but he was also a friend, and I knew I could share with him that something wicked this way had come.

After we spent an afternoon together and I shared my situation, Pastor Dickow invited me to church that evening, where, as God would have it, Pastor Dickow was speaking on healing. Was this a coincidence? Not hardly. It was a God moment. So I went to church and listened to the message, only this time I listened more intently than I ever had before. I hung on every word. I even took notes.

At the end of the service, Pastor Dickow invited anyone who wanted to receive healing to come to the altar. I went. At that moment, I was totally willing to expose myself to the world and admit I had a problem. It can be a tough thing to be a Christian and have a conversation with someone about being sick. Let's linger on this for a moment.

When I discovered I was sick, I did not want anyone to know. When the symptoms arose, I did not want to talk about them, even after they stuck around. I felt as if I was less than a man. Seriously. This will be helpful to women reading this who are trying to understand the men in their lives and their reaction to their illness. When a man is sick, he feels weak. Men are supposed to wear bearskin rugs, beat our chests, and shout the victory cry. I don't care if you are seven feet tall like my man from the Congo or if you are four foot two and wear a wig like my laundromat guy—men want to be seen as Mel Gibson playing William Wallace in *Braveheart* (perhaps wearing something other than a kilt).

I did not want my wife to know I was sick. I did not want my children to know I was sick. And by all means, I did not want my peers, who were some of the most prominent faith-based leaders in the world, to know I was sick. I had already seen what illness can produce in the field I worked in as I served valiantly side-by-side with my father when he was fighting cancer.

This is not an indictment against the field where my vocation lies. My perception is based partly on my father's perception when he was dying and partly on the reality I saw and experienced firsthand as I walked the secret journey with him.

In some circles of the world of faith, especially the old-religion type, to be sick is to suggest that there is something wrong in your life spiritually. People can be quite judgmental at times. It is true that sickness and disease can indeed be the result of something going on in your life from a moral perspective, where you have opened a gateway to a demonic force and thus allowed sickness to prevail. But that is not always the case. Everyone who is sick does not need deliverance. Everyone who is sick is not sick as a result of living some secret life where sin abounds. Nevertheless, in old-time religion, the world in which my father was born and raised, the idea that sickness could be caused by something other than a spiritual shortcoming was not popular.

But that night in Chicago, I did not care about any of that. I was tired of being sick. I was getting my answer, and I knew God had it for me through Pastor Dickow.

I went to the altar and waited. Pastor Dickow was praying for everyone in that line. I looked around and saw the faces: men and women crying, waiting, hoping, and most importantly, believing. Pastor Dickow made it clear in his message that healing is already ours. It was given the moment Christ died at Calvary. This was not a big, bold prayers moment—this was receiving time; this was surrender time. I was there to surrender and to receive. Pastor Dickow finally made his way to me, and the prayer was a simple one. I did not feel any power shoot through my body, there was no heat sensation, I did not fall out in the Spirit, and I saw no visions. Pastor Dickow laid his hands on me, and he told me what the promises of God were, that God loved me and His grace was sufficient for me, and that I simply needed to believe it. In that moment my belief was at an all-time high. Pastor Dickow told me to "thank God for what He's already done in you." I did just that, and when I tell you that the next morning I woke to a pain-free, inflammation-free day, I am not exaggerating. With a clear heart and a sober mind, logically and without reservation, I am telling you that God healed me that day.

But if God healed me, then why the need for a journey? Is this book about the journey before the altar, and the altar experience was the answer? No. And here is where the rubber met the road.

Chapter 2

HEALED OR CURED?

A CCORDING TO THE medical establishment, *curing* means "eliminating all evidence of disease." The very definition suggests that sickness has a risk of coming back. And even though billions of dollars are spent on finding a cure to the litany of diseases that plague humanity, they continue to find themselves battling the symptoms war.

THE DEFINITION OF CURE

"I don't heal; that's all on you." A doctor actually told me that when I asked him if he could heal me. I used the word *heal* because that is the term we Christians use.

Doctors search for a cure, which in essence means "the end of your medical condition." But the truth is that the cure, as defined by the medical profession, often never truly manifests in the body of the one seeking it. *Cure* means "remission." *Cure* means "it is gone for a while." *Cure* means "the symptoms are gone." But *cure* in the language of God means "healed, gone completely, gone and never coming back; the root problem has been identified and addressed."

Almost all of the ten million doctors on the planet (as reported by World Health Organization figures)[1] are trained to diagnose and treat symptoms rather than to cure, to identify and address the root problem of what is causing sickness. Despite all the money spent by the government, major corporations, and nonprofits to find a cure, all we see is an entire industry geared toward the treatment of symptoms. Hardly anyone in the waiting room at medical offices across America goes back, sits on the cold, paper-draped table, and then experiences a real, deep-down discussion with the doctor on how to address the root of what is causing us to be so sick.

So we are going to delve into how God cures, because no one else can.

Doctors are not trained to deal with the root cause of illness and disease. And this is where the rubber actually meets the road when we are dealing with *cure* versus *heal*. We already discussed two definitions of *cure*—the medical establishment's definition and God's definition. We are going to add some more definitions to the mix. For our purposes, we are going to step away from the traditional Christian understanding of healing and define *healing* as "the process by which the body is restored at a cellular level" and *heal* as "to make well temporarily."

Doctors are trained to diagnose and treat symptoms. It was this truth that I had to get my head around before anything else and one that you must understand when starting this journey to discover that only God cures. So let's make it very clear.

To cure, according to medicine, is to pause something in your genes that is being expressed as symptoms through medication, surgery, or some other form of medical treatment. There is no guarantee that the illness is gone forever.

Healing, the process by which the body is restored at a cellular level, happens at the core. Healing happens at the root, dealing with cells, dealing with genes. It involves overcoming fear, dealing with guilt, moving past shame, learning to forgive, seeing yourself as God sees you, and taking dominion. Healing is the process that can eventually lead to a cure the way God defines it, with sickness eradicated completely.

The medical establishment cannot deliver an ounce of anything that I just described as necessary for curing you. The real cure, the God cure, will not happen inside the medical establishment; it will happen outside it. Treatment and management of symptoms and pain can happen inside the system of medicine. You follow the advice of your doctor (natural or conventional) to treat the surface problem, but the strategy to wage war on the root causes of illness and disease is going to be an outside-of-the-box battle.

God cures. He cures through opening the door to understanding, and our road to repair, recovery, and restoration begins when we take the responsibility to put into action something that only He can do at the very foundation of where sickness and disease began.

Knowledge is power, but knowledge without action is just information. Faith is dead without an agreement from us that works must be involved.

We must understand that there is no magic pill that will wipe out what is going on in your body. You may have been to the doctor over twenty times hoping for the right diagnosis, hoping that the next change in medication will be the perfect cocktail to make things right, but you are on the wrong track. That road leads to unnecessary tests, unnecessary procedures, and medications that will kill you slowly. You may feel helpless, but the reason for that is your hope is in the wrong place. Doctors can treat your symptoms, but they cannot truly cure what you have—because what you have starts with you.

Each and every doctor I saw to address the autoimmune disease that plagued my body talked about treatment, not how to eradicate it from my body. They wanted to medicate it, to help control it. My grandmother was diabetic. Her body did not make enough insulin to get glucose into her cells, where it was needed for her to live a balanced life. Her doctors treated her with insulin injections and medication to prop her up, never once looking deeper to attack the source of her disease. They were not on the mission to cure. They treated her to attempt to help her regain some normalcy to her life. The industry declares there is no cure for diabetes. My grandmother, a praying woman who was full of faith, died taking injections of insulin.

I did not understand the process of being made truly whole and that it required more than just a spiritual experience for me at the altar. I know that God's grace is sufficient. His love is unmerited. There is nothing that I can do to earn God's favor. He did it all at the cross.

But here are the facts: I was not cured; I was not whole. I experienced some improvement in my body, but sickness returned with a fury. God wanted to do more, down at the cellular level, by my putting my entire focus on Him and committing my body and my ways to Him. But none of that occurred. I stood, declared healing (the traditional kind), and walked away. This pattern is so textbook. As a result, we break down and run back to medicine, as if medicine is our cure. Thus, the body of Christ is riddled with sickness and disease. Those with the biggest names are getting sick and living in limitation and loneliness, and some are dying right before our very eyes. We are talking about men and women of great faith.

BEYOND THE SURFACE

It has been many years since I was first told I was sick. It has been not quite as many years since I stood in front of Pastor Dickow and he prayed for my healing. Pastor Dickow did his job, and he did it well. God did His job, and He did it well. I didn't do mine. I treated God like the medical establishment treats finding a cure. It skims the surface. We pop a pill. We go back to our normal lives, which got us sick in the first place.

So what actually happened when I went to the altar?

I was treated. Pastor Dickow meant for me to receive my "healing," but it was really where I would begin the journey of change—change in my thinking, change in my living. Pastor Dickow was directing me to allow God to change me from the inside out. Because I did not understand what needed to happen in me, meaning I was not ready to commit to change anything that led to my condition, I was not going for healing—I was going for treatment.

Treatment is what happens after you cut yourself. You clean the wound. You put on some salve. The area of the body becomes inflamed, which means that blood rushes to the area of the injury, and the process of healing begins. Parents understand this process of treatment to help the body heal itself. When our child falls riding his bike and skins a knee, we clean the wound and put on a Band-Aid, and in a couple days all that's left is a scab. The body does what it was designed to do; we aid the process as we can and expect healing to happen.

But if a child falls off his bike every day, do we just shrug it off as clumsy, or do we stop, think deeply, and work to find the reason why he cannot seem to pedal without falling? Is our child going to end up with a broken bone or a permanent head injury that a Band-Aid won't fix? We are suddenly moving beyond treatment and searching for a cure, a way to identify and address the root issue that goes way beyond a skinned knee.

So what do we do? Do we put the training wheels back on? Do we install a governor on the bike so that it cannot go past ten miles per hour? Do we cover our child in protective gear before every bike ride? No! But that is exactly what the definition of *cure* is in the medical profession. Medicate it and treat it without addressing the root cause.

The parent of a child who continually falls off his bike is going to slow down and figure out why the fall is happening in the first place. Does the child need more training? Perhaps the seat or handlebars need adjustment. We get to the source. We go down deep. We get to the root of the issue to fix it once and for all.

God's cure is the end of your medical condition, your financial situation, your relationship problem, and more. God's cure is a process to eradicate the problem completely. He wants to completely remove what is in your system, your body, that caused you to become sick and diseased. He wants you to be restored, renewed, and whole.

> Do not lie to one another, seeing that you have put off the old self with its practices and have put on the new self, which is being renewed in knowledge after the image of its creator.
>
> —COLOSSIANS 3:9–10, ESV

That, in reference to your former manner of life, you lay aside the old self, which is being corrupted in accordance with the lusts of deceit, and that you be renewed in the

spirit of your mind, and put on the new self, which in the
likeness of God has been created in righteousness and holi-
ness of the truth.

—EPHESIANS 4:22–24, NASB

God has used medicine many, many times to bring healing.
But what we want is a cure, when a disease has been completely
eradicated with no possibility of ever coming back. With God
this is possible.

If we do not understand what sickness really is, where it comes
from, or what caused us to get sick, then it will be like those who
have had cancer and achieve remission, but the cancer inevitably
returns. And when it comes back, it comes back with a fury. The
Bible says, "When an impure spirit comes out of a person, it goes
through arid places seeking rest and does not find it. Then it says,
'I will return to the house I left.' When it arrives, it finds the
house unoccupied, swept clean and put in order. Then it goes
and takes with it seven other spirits more wicked than itself, and
they go in and live there. And the final condition of that person
is worse than the first. That is how it will be with this wicked
generation" (Matt. 12:43–45, NIV).

EPIGENETICS

When you get sick, when you are diagnosed with something the
medical establishment says is incurable, you get really serious
about finding truth, which can mean refusing to go the way of
popular thinking.

What I believe is this: when sin entered the scene, each one of
us from was sick the womb. We were born into this world sick
at our core, down deep at the cellular, genetic, and DNA levels.

Science is proving what I am saying. The field of study is called
epigenetics.

Like that talking box I told you about in the last chapter, technology has finally caught up with the insatiable need for humanity to understand the mysteries of the universe. It's funny actually. In Ephesians 3, God told humanity that the mysteries of Christ would be fulfilled in the fullness of time. Romans 11:36 says, "For of Him and through Him and to Him are all things." And if we, His creation, are of Him, and if our spirits, our souls, and even our bodies, our health, and our genetic makeup are subject to Him, here we are on the timeline of all eternity, experiencing God's way of giving us a glimpse into His great laboratory of creation.

Some discoveries are nothing short of unbelievable. Discoveries in genetics alone are availing us better medicine and, like the Six Million Dollar Man of the late 1970s, we are finding ways to be stronger, be faster, and in many cases live longer. After all, there was a time in history when man lived to over nine hundred years old. (See Genesis 5.) Then suddenly, for reasons explained in Genesis, God cut us to one hundred and twenty years on earth. But who even lives to one hundred and twenty? Many will soon enough. The most exhilarating thing in terms of modern discovery is our ability to treat disease and how we can improve life. Consider that we are now cloning sheep and growing replacement body parts, and stem cell research is garnering a lot of attention.[2] As science races to learn more, they realize even more how little they know.

However, it seems that we are getting sicker than ever before and at a younger age. We are living longer than we did in, say, the Dark Ages. Nevertheless, it seems that early sickness is sweeping children across the globe and that debilitating sickness and disease is on the rise all over the world: arthritis in its more than one hundred different forms; diabetes in its multiple types; and cancer, cancer, and more cancer. It has been said that every single one of us will have someone in our immediate family or extended family circle hit with the wretchedness of cancer in our lifetime. I have seen it three times in my circle in the last ten years alone.

And sickness is not limited to the physical. Mental illness in its many forms is purportedly on the rise.[3] There's depression, bipolar disorder, and anxiety and stress disorders. But hey, sick is sick, no matter how you slice it. Mild illness will cause minor discomfort and inconvenience, whereas severe or progressive diseases can ravage the very core of one's existence, causing long-term effects. And depression is real. It can paralyze you and trap you. It is a lonely place to live.

But science has discovered something and given it a name: epigenetics. It is sweeping conventional and non-conventional medicine faster than anything we have ever seen before.

Let's break the word down. *Epi*, the prefix, comes from the Greek and means "upon, besides, attached to, and over."[4] *Genetics* means "the study of genes." And what are genes? No, not Levi's! Maybe you hear someone talk about genes and think about what caused you to have your dad's nose or your mom's toes. We hear, "Oh, my hair's going early because I got my grandpa's genes." But there's more and a much deeper need to understand what genes really are and what they do.

A gene is "a region of DNA that encodes function."[5] Genes are what make up heredity and are made up of DNA. Our genes are commonly around twenty-seven thousand base pairs long, but they can be up to two million.[6] And science discovered that we have over twenty thousand genes. We have two copies of each one of those genes.[7]

Let me try and summarize the breakdown simply. Your body is made up of cells. Inside your cells you have nucleotides—over three billion of them to be exact—and these nucleotides have over twenty thousand genes, which form twenty-three pairs of chromosomes. You got half of each pair of chromosomes from your father and half from your mother.[8]

These chromosomes are, in essence, what determined what you look like. But according to what epigenetics is saying, genes influence so much more. I'll get into that in a second.

According to its definition, a symptom is "a sign of a disease or illness." Symptoms of a cold, for example, include nasal congestion and a cough. So if you are displaying those symptoms, you are considered symptomatic. *Symptomatic* means "showing symptoms of something."[9] What you are showing symptoms of exists at a cellular level, at a DNA level, and is expressed by your genes. And watch this: whatever symptoms I have were directly passed to me from those before me. Somehow, someway, I triggered their activation. Or said another way, something caused the sickness and disease that lay sleeping and lurking inside me to be switched on.

But how can that be true? What about that scripture in Jeremiah that says, "'For I know the plans I have for you,' declares the LORD, 'plans to prosper you and not to harm you, plans to give you hope and a future'" (Jer. 29:11, NIV)? Or what about Jeremiah 1:5: "Before I formed you in the womb I knew you; before you were born I sanctified you; I ordained you a prophet to the nations"? God hasn't changed His mind. So what's going on?

As I continued to study, I discovered I was not alone in being sick. Almost everyone on earth is sick at a cellular level.[10] Many just haven't expressed the symptoms yet. According to a 2013 study published in *The Lancet*, 95 percent of the world's population had an illness or injury![11] I'm visual, so let's look at it this way: There are a hundred people at your house for a party. Only five of them will make it through the year without being sick.

We know about the prevalence of illnesses such as cancer,

heart disease and other cardiovascular issues, arthritis, and autoimmune diseases, but there are other health issues affecting millions of people, such as skin diseases, mental illness and developmental disorders, digestive system issues, and diabetes.[12]

What? How are we sick? What is happening? Where is it coming from?

It is so confusing out there. Out where? In the land of what do I eat, what shouldn't I eat, how do I get healthy, how do I avoid getting sick, how do I lose twenty pounds. The "fact" that we use only 10 percent of the brain, for example, is a myth.[13] Seriously, it is. We've all heard it, and you've likely repeated it, but it's not true.

In truth, who hasn't heard and shared an amazing fact only to find out later on it was bogus? How about the one about apples: "An apple a day keeps the doctor away." Not true either. Completely overstated. Apples are loaded with vitamin C and fiber, both of which can help with long-term health, but an apple, like other fruits, loads our cells with sugar, and sugar can kill you slowly.[14]

One day you are getting up, getting dressed, running out the door to take the kids to school, rushing to get to the office, and grabbing a banana to jump start a healthy day, believing that it's great for you. And then the next time you boot up your laptop, you get hit with an article that reveals bananas can be bad for you too.[15]

When I was growing up, the TV commercials told me to drink milk. It was good for me. Then the experts told me that dairy was bad for me.[16] At one point eating margarine was the only way toast would taste good, but I was told to stay away from the other creamy stuff because that would clog my arteries. Then we find out that butter is actually the healthier choice, and margarine should be used for greasing plane parts.[17] I am exaggerating a little, but my point is made and not too far from the truth.

We are sick. We are all unhealthy, and in truth, much of how we got here did not happen overnight, and it isn't all your fault. The truth is, it's all confusing. In fact, it was designed to be confusing. There is without question a hand at play, a puppet master behind the scenes working to keep everything mixed up, confused, and out of whack.

So whose fault is it then? Well, we are not going to blame that burger chain for asking you if you wanted to supersize that or the advertising agencies for making things that are bad for you look healthy. We are not going to jump on the conspiracy wagon that the big pharmaceutical companies are behind it all. Nearly all those characters are suspects in what I call "the grand delusion," but they are not the wizard behind the curtain.

Epigenetics speaks to signs, traits, symptoms, or changes—an actual, physical mark on our DNA when someone has survived an important experience, whether it's positive or negative. These marks actually alter the function of genes.[18] Did you get that? Simply put, tragedy, suffering, great and prolonged stress, and experiences in life we survived by enduring and hanging on to the altar have affected the behavior of our genes, have actually altered regions of our DNA, and suddenly sickness and disease have been switched on!

But it does not stop with just our personal experiences. It is also what we are exposed to, our surroundings. Epigenetics is telling us that what happens in the womb affects our genes. Yes. Inside the womb we are exposed to environmental toxins, stress from your mother and what she went through when you were inside her, the good stuff and the bad stuff. When you come out into the light, psychological stress, adversity, poverty, abuse, etc. all factor in way down deep inside of you, in the genes that God created to function a certain way, to express power, to express what He created you to do in this world.

Epigenetics is not just sweeping medicine; it is an emerging field in consciousness because they are actually discovering that in addition to sickness and disease markers, genes pass along memory, fear, depression, anxiety, low self-confidence, and even darker traits from generations past.[19]

If there were ever a case for confirmation of scriptures such as Deuteronomy 5:9, "visiting the iniquity of the fathers upon the children to the third and fourth generations," it is the discoveries of epigenetics. And if there were ever an argument for a super-natural demonic force at work, it would likewise be confirmed by the discovery of science.

Somehow I uncovered the truth. I asked God to reveal to me why I was sick. I asked Him to heal me, and I received healing but only temporarily. I then looked deeper, wanting to under-stand what sickness really was, and I got the medical definition. I sought to understand why it was plaguing humanity and why medicine and technology could not seem to cure it. We needed more than just healing of a wound. Band-Aids just don't last.

There had to be more. I had to find the cure—God's cure. God had not allowed me to endure pain and struggle for so long for no reason. He told me to look deeper, to ask why.

I have interviewed some of the greatest minds in medi-cine, health and wellness, physics, technology, spirituality, and divinity. I have crossed continents. I have been to Africa and to the remote jungles of Central and South America. I have been to the highest mountains. I have been to the holy places, to the caves of the prophets. What I discovered was a secret diabolical plot of the enemy right beneath our noses. And in discovering what Satan was really up to, I found out how God cures.

Chapter 3

THE GRAND DELUSION

I HAVE CALLED THIS chapter The Grand Delusion because I want you to understand the truth about this journey to healing and wholeness. This is a truth that should be in neon lights as the very first thing we see when our eyes open after we leave the womb, when we emerge into the light and into this thing called life. We are going to start by repeating what we have learned about God cures.

It starts with understanding that when we get sick, we tend to go to the same source for eradication of the illness—the conventional medical establishment. Some have become wise to and understand the importance of non-conventional, alternative, natural wellness practices.

In either case, we are seeking an eradication of sickness, and yet neither industry can offer it for many illnesses that are reported as incurable. Our cure, the complete healing at the root cause of illness, likely is not going to come from an outside source. The external entities of conventional medicine are in the business of treating and managing symptoms and driving illness into remission.

Only God can cure in the way that I describe in this book because God's strategy, found in the Word, focuses completely on bringing wholeness to our misaligned, fractured lives and fractured selves, centering on the eradication of what has caused us to become sick—the root problems in our internal man, spirit, soul, and body. Everything else outside of us is treatment. Everything else is temporary.

Merriam-Webster defines *cure* as "recovery or relief from a disease."[1] God's definition is more akin to what we find in 2 Chronicles 7:14, which is "restoration and deliverance of the afflicted land": "If My people who are called by My name will humble themselves, and pray and seek My face, and turn from their wicked ways, then I will hear from heaven, and will forgive their sin and heal their land."

God cures. Medicine cures nothing. Medicine might eradicate a parasite or a virus and call it curing; however, conventional medicine does not teach us how to avoid or fortify us against the virus or parasite, so we might get it all over again. If fractures in the total composition of a person remain, sickness will inevitably return.

There is, simply, a conspiracy at play. Better stated, there is a war raging at you, against you, and within you to steal, to kill, and to destroy you and the future God intended for you. And the great orchestrator of this whole thing has a name. Keep in mind that according to God's Word, while the secret things belong to God, the things that are revealed belong to us (Deut. 29:29).

THE ORCHESTRATOR

In order for you to fully understand where I am taking you on this journey, to be able to see it for what it really is, I am going to have to take you back in time—way back in time, at the start of Creation, before Adam and Eve, way before the Cross, somewhere in Genesis around the time of what some call the gap theory, and before we see Satan appearing on the scene in Genesis 3:1.

Satan is a created being and did not exist "in the beginning." God, like a great painter with a white canvas, created the heavens and the earth. The Creator set into motion everything we see, touch, feel, or smell. And after God set everything into motion and designed the order of things, He created Satan and called him by name. The original Hebrew, *satan*, means "an opponent, an adversary, withstand, or oppose,"[2] as found in verses such as Numbers 22:22.

Understand that God did not create anything evil, not even the devil. The devil (also known as Lucifer, Satan, the fallen son of the dawn or morning of Isaiah 14:12, and the accuser of the brethren of Revelation 12:10) was actually created perfect in his original state. You may find that hard to believe, but it is a fact.

> You were the seal of perfection, full of wisdom and perfect in beauty. You were in Eden, the garden of God... You were the anointed cherub who covers; I established you; you were on the holy mountain of God... You were perfect in your ways from the day you were created, till iniquity was found in you.
>
> —EZEKIEL 28:12–15

The definition of *iniquity* is not simply "sin." It is "grossly unfair behavior."[3] Keep reading from Ezekiel:

By the abundance of your trading you became filled with violence within, and you sinned; therefore I cast you as a profane thing out of the mountain of God; and I destroyed you, O covering cherub, from the midst of the fiery stones. Your heart was lifted up because of your beauty; you corrupted your wisdom for the sake of your splendor; I cast you to the ground, I laid you before kings, that they might gaze at you. You defiled your sanctuaries by the multitude of your iniquities, by the iniquity of your trading; therefore I brought fire from your midst; it devoured you, and I turned you to ashes upon the earth in the sight of all who saw you. All who knew you among the peoples are astonished at you; you have become a horror, and shall be no more forever.

—EZEKIEL 28:16–19

So way back somewhere in the beginning, God created everything, including the grand orchestrator of intent for man's demise, Satan. I will not take the time to tell you the whole story, but many of us know it from growing up in the church—how the devil was consumed with pride and thought he could jockey for a position of power above God, and the created was ejected by the Creator. And by the way, a little trivia point for those who love theology: his name was Lucifer in heaven; he became Satan when he was cast out.

The Book of Revelation tells us, "And war broke out in heaven: Michael and his angels fought with the dragon; and the dragon and his angels fought, but they did not prevail, nor was a place found for them in heaven any longer. So the great dragon was cast out, that serpent of old, called the Devil and Satan, who deceives the whole world; he was cast to the earth, and his angels were cast out with him" (Rev. 12:7–9). It is at this moment, when the one created with a seal of perfection but consumed with himself and with pride is literally thrown out of heaven to the earth, that it all really goes crazy for mankind.

The Bible tells us that when Satan was kicked out of heaven, he went to the earth. He roams free. He is not in chains. The angels who fell with him are in chains (2 Pet. 2:4; Jude 1:6), but Satan is free to roam. Now is not the time to try to explain why exactly. For now, just know that Satan is around, roaming free and seeking to mess you up.

First Peter 5:8 reads, "Be of sober spirit, be on the alert. Your adversary, the devil, prowls around like a roaring lion, seeking someone to devour" (NASB). This is where it gets real. God placed Adam in the garden. He created him, and He put him there. We are going to come back to Adam in the garden in a moment because it is important.

PERFECTLY CREATED

We now know that there is intelligent design behind our universe, not to mention the other theoretical universes science suggests exist outside of our own universe. Scientists can tell us how things move and their chemical composition, but they cannot tell us what set it all in motion. They do believe, however, that what exists is far too complex, too perfectly organized and arranged, and working together too harmoniously to be just happenstance. We are talking about millions of stars and the planets spinning in perfect order and in perfect position in relation to the sun. Is this luck? No way. It is the perfect order of the perfect One who created it all, God. And the One who is omnipotent, omniscient, and capable of creation with such perfection also created man— our spirits, our souls, and our physical bodies, our bodies being the dwelling place of our spirits and souls. Consider the majesty and power of the Creator who created it all. God set it all into motion.

I believe that science and technology are catching up to reveal what God did, not what evolution did. If we can agree with anything relative to change over time, it would be that God created living things to adapt. If I could help the theorists understand how to explain what they see when they look at how organic, biological matter changes over time, it's that—adaptation. But adaptation based upon environmental conditions does not change God's plan for creation and everything that is created "according to its kind." (See Genesis 1.) Science clearly reveals that there is a God. And now because of science and technology, we can see that beneath the skin there are trillions of cells within our bodies containing our DNA, our genes. So we have trillions of microscopic moving parts, perfectly organized for perfect function, that carry intelligence. In fact, *cell* comes from the Greek word *cella*, meaning "small rooms."[4] Our cells are like tiny rooms that have intelligence and carry the information by which we function as a created thing.

Adam was placed in a perfect garden with perfect conditions to protect a perfectly created being. And then, somewhere before Genesis 3, Lucifer was expelled from heaven, becoming Satan, and through a series of unfortunate events Adam sinned and lost his place in a perfect garden created for a perfect being—a being who was supposed to live forever. Adam was expelled from the place of perfection, and he was then subject and susceptible to contamination—to sickness and disease.

Adaptation over time has not changed the fact that the genes that were in Adam are in us. The same genes that were designed to function in a place of perfection now operate in us. Only now, since sin came on the scene and man's spirit died, those genes are susceptible to disunity, fracture, exposure, and adaptation to an environment that is not perfect. Those genes, as science proves, now malfunction. And unless those malfunctions are handled God's way, according to His plan for man's reconciliation to Him, the impact will be felt for generations to come.

God's creative, created order of things has not changed. God created our cells to function a certain way. He created our genes, programmed with specific functions to tell the DNA what to do. How you were built, how your genes were built to function, and how your genes were encoded with function are connected to the place where Adam was intended to reside—a perfect place of order.

But now let's consider something. Who else understands how God set everything into motion and created everything, including man? Jesus? Yes. The Spirit of God? Of course. We were made in their image. But do you know who else understands how we were created? Lucifer.

We already mentioned his pride. He was unable to accept his place in the created order, to accept his rank and file. He believed that he could rise above God, so he was literally thrown out of heaven. The Bible calls him "the prince of the power of the air" (Eph. 2:2), meaning he currently is at work here on the earth.

Satan sits back and says, "Hey, fallen angelic hosts who rolled out with me! Did you see how God made these guys? Humans? Were you there when He said, 'Let Us make man in Our image, according to Our likeness'? Did you see that? Did you hear that? Did you see how He created them? They've got all these trillions of cells."

Satan gets it. Satan is looking beneath the hood, looking beneath our skin. He is not human, he was not created like we were, and he does not have God's image, God's power. But Satan does have the blueprint that tells him how we were made. He has the blueprint that tells him how we function. He has the blueprint that gives him the instructions on how to mess us up at a cellular level. He cannot create anything because he does not have that power, but he understands creation and has the ability to influence its disruption.

At the moment when God said man's years would only be one hundred and twenty on the earth (Gen. 6:3), I believe Satan heard it too. But we do not fully understand what Satan heard. Satan heard that decay, cellular death was possible. We have forgotten that Satan understands physics, he understands biology, and he understands chemistry. Again, he does not have the power to create, but he completely understands creation and how it works.

PROGRAMMED IN YOUR GENES

Science has discovered that our genes have our hair color, eye color, height, personality traits, and even memory programmed into them.[5] But Satan knows that also programmed into our genes are traits of sickness and disease from generations past. He also knows that these markers lie dormant but may be awakened by conditions of the environment.

Stress, heartbreak, job loss, tragedy, divorce—just make a list of the things that have tormented you, fractured you, and caused sleepless nights, the things you thought you had worked through and recovered from, the things you thought you had survived and overcome, the things you went to the altar and prayed about and got the victory. These are all things in our environment that affect us.

What you may not know is that all these things, which are all part of the plan Satan set up to derail your life, were not just about getting you to take your eyes off Jesus. I believe that Satan was attempting to manipulate your DNA by fracturing your spirit and soul and thereby turning on the switch in your genes to express sickness and disease in your body!

Listen to me: Satan is not in control of your body. It does not belong to him. He has no jurisdiction over it. He lacks what God has the power to do—to create. He cannot go into your body and flip on the switch, but he can put you in a position and subject you to fractures of your total composition so that the switch can be turned on by itself.

This is what science has discovered, and it is called epigenetics. But it is not just about disease. They are discovering that what you are exposed to as a child can turn this switch on also.[6] Have you ever wondered why they say alcoholics have a disease? If one of your parents was an alcoholic, then you as their child are susceptible to the same. This is gene expression—the process by which DNA instructions are turned into functions. I am reaching here, but it almost seems that adulterers also produce adulterers, liars produce liars, gamblers beget gamblers, and abusers beget abusers. How much is learned and how much is gene expression because Satan orchestrated circumstances that led to the flipping of the switch? Psychologists, psychotherapists, doctors, and scientific researchers are now exploring how something that existed in two generations past has memory and markers programmed into the DNA that has been passed along.[7]

This says to me that if Satan knew that the negative markers could be triggered, he must also know that the positive, God-created, and predestined kingdom gifts can also be triggered and expressed through these genetic markers, which Satan would perceive as a danger.

As I look back at my own family line, I see a pattern. Did Satan know that Ray Davis, my father, would be gifted to preach? He would have known it if he made the connection that Ray's father and his father before him were also preachers. And consider:

every one of those men also died from heart disease by their late fifties.

We say things like, "Oh, she's just like her mother," or, "He's just like his grandfather," but we have no idea about the reality of what we just said. We have no idea how real it is. This is part of the grand delusion I am talking about; we have placed the responsibility solely on the people.

Yes, we are responsible for our actions, but we have put an overwhelming amount of responsibility on the sons and daughters of the Most High God to make it through, to overcome, to avoid bad decisions, when all the while we did not even realize that something greater than just our right decisions is actually at play. There is influence and stuff happening at a cellular level in our DNA that is driving us in one direction or another from the inside.

Here is the revelation: just as Satan knows that markers for destruction reside in your genes, he also knows that God placed gifts, talents, purpose, and destiny there. That is what Satan is after. That is what he is afraid of being expressed.

There is a war being waged inside of us. Since Satan cannot get inside of those of us who are saved and covered by the blood of Jesus, he has to find a way to initiate gene expression that can wreak havoc through sickness or disease so that the kingdom power never finds its way into his domain.

Let me provide a disclaimer here, lest you think I am trying to dispute a body of Christian theology and study in generational curses. I do believe in the biblical concept of generational curses. I believe that Satan's minions are at work in our generational lines. They are observant of the vices and failures of our forefathers, and they work in the shadows to bring out these familiar downfalls in life. How is it that entire groups of people can struggle with the same difficulties year after year, generation after generation, no matter how much information, training, or culture they receive? It is because demonic spirits are on the loose, and they use what is familiar to trip us up.

As I said earlier, I believe that the science of epigenetics is confirming what Scripture says. Take the example of the sin of lying by both Abraham and his son Isaac. Genesis 20 records that Abraham lied to King Abimelech about his wife, Sarah, calling her his sister. This clearly occurred before the birth of Isaac, which was recorded in Genesis 21. Genesis 26 records that Isaac (after the death of Abraham) lied to a different King Abimelech about his wife, Rebekah, calling her his sister.

It was not socialization that caused Isaac to repeat the sin of his father; Isaac was not alive when Abraham lied about Sarah. Isaac did not learn of this pattern by observation. Yet both men blamed fear as their motivator. When Abimelech asked Abraham why he lied, Abraham said, "Because I thought, surely the fear of God is not in this place; and they will kill me on account of my wife" (Gen. 20:11).

When the men of Gerar asked Isaac about his wife, the Scripture tells us that "he said, 'She is my sister'; for he was afraid to say, 'She is my wife,' because he thought, 'lest the men of the place kill me for Rebekah, because she is beautiful to behold'" (Gen. 26:7).

Abraham thought. Isaac thought. I believe strongly that demonic spirits whispered these internal thoughts of fear and intimidation to Abraham and Isaac.

THE REVELATION OF EPIGENETICS

Epigenetics provides the revelation on how these curses are being activated! And that is where the revelation comes to us. Satan only has to initiate the curses that are already in our genes.

However, we are free moral agents, covered by the blood, and saved because Jesus died for us at Calvary, and God cannot undo what He created. In other words, God is so just, is so true, and has such integrity that He will not undo how He created man to function. Sin abounds, but God will not undo what sin can cause in our mortal bodies—or how our genes will respond. It's like this: God creates a Bentley. He says it functions a certain way, and He provides the owner's manual. If you operate the vehicle according to the manual, it will produce the outcome He said was made possible by its design. And yet despite having the owner's manual, you treat the vehicle like a Yugo. We do the same thing with our bodies.

Satan knows he must initiate the expression of what lies dormant in our genes so the switch will flip itself on. Once the switch is flipped, our personalities begin to warp. We become angry, bitter, frustrated, pessimistic, anxious, double-minded, sick, and diseased. This downward spiral is a vicious one. Satan has determined that all he has to do to keep from us the gifts and callings we were meant to express is to give us one good nudge, and down we go.

Myles Munroe said, "The wealthiest places in the world are not gold mines, oil fields, diamond mines or banks. The wealthiest place is the cemetery. There lies companies that were never started, masterpieces that were never painted...In the cemetery there is buried the greatest treasure of untapped potential. There is a treasure within you that must come out. Don't go to the grave with your treasure still within you." [8]

If Satan can orchestrate the flipping of the switch in your parents, then he initiates tragedy, chaos, and destruction even in their bloodline; the memory and markers will be programmed in their genes to be expressed in their DNA and also in yours. That is the business Satan is in. Satan is not in the business of putting stuff together. He is in the business of tearing stuff apart. The Bible says he is a roaring lion, seeking someone to devour (1 Pet. 5:8). He is the author of chaos. He is trying to flip the switch on genes, knowing that if he can initiate chaos in the children, then those children will reproduce the same chaos in their children.

Little did we realize that the bad decisions we make do not just impact our lives, but we are setting up a predisposition for bad decisions in the lives of our children. All of this, what I call the grand delusion, the sickness and disease, is Satan's weapon to steal from us the expression of our gifts, our talents, and our discovery of the purpose and destiny God planned for our lives.

It's about chaos. What Satan did in heaven, what he did in the garden, he is attempting to do inside of you. But God tells us what the end of the story is. It is found in the Book of Revelation. Satan knows that his time is limited. He knows the end of the story too.

You see, Satan is not really interested in us. He is consumed by us. There is a difference. If he can mess us up, ruin our lives, and stop our gifts and calling from being expressed, he believes that he in turn will disrupt the plan of heaven.

Rest assured that will never happen. But the war plan is obvious. What God has built, Satan attempts to destroy. God creates, and Satan tries to corrupt. This isn't even about us. We are just in the crossfire.

But listen, there is an answer. There is hope. The end of the story has yet to come. While there is breath, there is hope. By the simple fact that you are reading this book, God is still working in you and for you. God's big plans for your future remain. No matter how bleak things appear, how black things look, how tired or how sick you may be, God is still the redeemer.

Satan believes that if he can move you into a place of sickness and disease, then just like the children of Israel, you will be trapped and in bondage, and the gifts, talents, calling, and purpose of God for your life will never see the light. The words found in Deuteronomy were true for the children of Israel, and they are true for you today: "Because the LORD loves you, and because He would keep the oath which He swore to your fathers, the LORD has brought you out with a mighty hand, and redeemed you from the house of bondage" (Deut. 7:8). The Bible tells us that the promises of God are yes and amen forever (2 Cor. 1:20). And the covenant that the Lord entered with us, His children, and the promises He made before we came into being are still alive and active for today.

So even though Satan is trying to keep us in bondage, God has created a way for us to overcome, to break free from the prison of sickness and disease and emerge as the greatest version of ourselves the world has ever known.

You see, I have another revelation from science and medicine also. The study of epigenetics tells us that just as you can flip the switch to express sickness and disease, your body has the ability to flip the switch off! God has created in you, by the works of His hands, the ability to flip the switch off. That's right. If the switch can be turned on, you can turn it off. By turning off the expression of bad stuff, by moving yourself into a place of peace, harmony, balance, and correct working order, you can push back the disease and begin to heal, fully and completely. And this, my dear friend, is why I embarked upon my journey to discover how God cures.

I have encapsulated my years of research and discovery into a twenty-one-day journey to arrest the markers of sickness and disease by identifying and addressing how you flipped them on in the first place. I have clearly laid out for you how to move your spirit, your soul, and your body into a place of alignment, because when that occurs, something remarkable happens.

We will start with showing you what Satan knows, which is how God made you. This is not just about your body. God made you in three parts, spirit, soul, and body. Your understanding of these three parts of you, of your makeup, of the total composition of you, will lead you on a journey to total and absolute healing and wholeness, at the core, from the inside out.

Psalm 111:9 reads, "He has sent redemption to His people; He has ordained His covenant forever; holy and awesome is His name" (NASB). Isaiah 62:12 tells us, "And they shall call them The Holy People, The Redeemed of the LORD; and you shall be called Sought Out, A City Not Forsaken."

Those precious words are true for you. The Lord has ordained His covenant forever. You are redeemed, and you will not be forsaken. Read on.

Chapter 4

THE TOTAL COMPOSITION OF YOU

THROUGH THE STUDY of epigenetics, we discovered how external influences of stress, strain, exposure to prolonged struggle, trauma, chemical toxins, and even polluted thoughts have fractured us and led to the evolution of sickness and disease in our bodies and minds. We have discovered that genes have memory, and that issues our parents struggled with, including addictive behaviors, personality disorders, alcoholism, adultery, and more, have in many cases been embedded within our DNA.

Now, understand this scientific evidence is not the same as "claiming" it, as some in the church may declare. Please do not fall victim to utter ignorance by ignoring what God, through scientific advancement and breakthrough technology, is doing to reveal to us the schemes of Satan! Our bodies were created to function a certain way. But when sin entered the scene, we were expelled from the perfect state found in the garden, and our bodies are therefore subject to epigenetic exposure.

This is fact, not fiction. To ignore the biological function and engineering of our body is to ignore the operational blueprint of its function revealed through science and technology. I believe God is completely behind these mysteries being revealed to us.

THE TEMPLE OF THE HOLY SPIRIT

Some in the body of Christ have looked at science, medicine, and technology as the enemy of the church for far too long. Theologians have skated by on scriptural interpretation, placing all the responsibility on the believer to exert some force of faith as the only measure to overcome illness. And when the healing never materialized, it became the burden and fault of the believer. Instead, we need to drill down on what is really going on in the body, searching for a true discovery of how the body works. By ignoring the working of the body, we are ignoring the laws of physics and biology. We have forgotten that actions cause reactions. We have dodged exercise, good nutrition, and other healthy habits only to find church leaders and laypeople alike with disease-ridden lives stemming from poor lifestyles, bad eating decisions, lack of exercise, lack of sleep, lack of hydration, and sugared diets, all leading to addictions, mental illness, abuse of the body, and cellular decay. Our pulpits are often populated by preachers who have become obese or nearly so; they have mastered the art of the sermon and song, but somewhere they lost their responsibility to be stewards of the temple of the Holy Spirit.

> Do you not know that your bodies are temples of the Holy Spirit, who is in you, whom you have received from God?

You are not your own; you were bought at a price. Therefore honor God with your bodies.

—1 CORINTHIANS 6:19–20, NIV

I urge you therefore, brothers, by the mercies of God, that you present your bodies as a living sacrifice, holy, and acceptable to God, which is your reasonable service of worship.

—ROMANS 12:1, MEV

By embracing insight and understanding of what medicine and science have proven to us about how our bodies function on the inside, and by learning what Satan knows, you conquer Satan's power over you. Knowledge is power. Before you began reading this book, Satan had insight and information you did not have yet about how your body functions. Therefore, Satan had the jump on you by having a complete understanding of the three parts of you—your total composition. By understanding your total composition, he was in a position of power to influence it. By influencing your surroundings, he was in fact fracturing your parts. He did this by simply bringing misalignment to the proper order and function of the parts of your makeup, which beckons sickness and disease to follow like a shadow.

This is logic. And to ignore logic is to suggest that God did not put the power of the brain in our heads to use. God expects us to use our minds, and this is a time for processing data, not simply practicing the power of positive thinking!

WONDER UPON WONDER

The New Testament tells us, "But someone who does not know, and then does something wrong, will be punished only lightly. When someone has been given much, much will be required in return; and when someone has been entrusted with much, even more will be required" (Luke 12:48, NLT). That is not judgment. It is actually good news. It means that while we are claiming and walking out our healing (in the traditional understanding of the word) and using our faith to stomp out scorpions, we are also tapping into a revelation that God has provided so we can be completely cured—not just healed and then fall back into the life that got us sick in the first place.

You may think this flies in the face of 1 Corinthians 1:19: "For it is written: 'I will destroy the wisdom of the wise; the intelligence of the intelligent I will frustrate'" (NIV). But does it really? Is God saying that we are not to understand the nature of the things He created? I don't think so. Look at the scripture that the apostle Paul is quoting: "Therefore once more I will astound these people with wonder upon wonder; the wisdom of the wise will perish, the intelligence of the intelligent will vanish" (Isa. 29:14, NIV). The word for *wonder* can mean "an extraordinary, hard to understand thing."[1]

I believe God is telling us something that is revelation. One "wonder" is what is available to us in the natural—the insight of science, biology, and the understanding of our physical makeup. Yet there is another wonder, "wonder upon wonder." The other "wonder" is the *supernatural*. It is that which cannot be understood by the wonder of the natural. You see, what is going to confound the wise is when we combine the power of what we can know naturally and ultimately what God does supernaturally!

If you are sick, there is full and complete eradication available through the power of God and through the information, knowledge, and understanding He is revealing to us through medicine and science.

THE THREE PARTS OF YOU

Let's start with understanding what the three parts of you really are and what their functions are. Through this understanding you will see that their proper function is affected by a proper order. By understanding the proper order of the three parts of the human composition, you will discover the scheme Satan has been concocting all along and how he has been winning on the battlefield of your mind. And you will learn how you are inflicting yourself with the onslaught of illness, thereby robbing yourself of the full discovery of your gift, your purpose, and how generations before you have been blinded to their destiny!

We find in the Scriptures that the first man ever made, Adam, was created perfect, and he was made in the image and likeness of God: "Then God said, 'Let Us make man in Our image, according to Our likeness; let them have dominion over the fish of the sea, over the birds of the air, and over the cattle, over all the earth and over every creeping thing that creeps on the earth'" (Gen. 1:26). If we bounce over to the Book of Luke, we find that Adam was even called the son of God: "The son of Enosh, the son of Seth, the son of Adam, the son of God" (Luke 3:38).

This is not hard to believe or understand. You know the story. Jesus was placed on the earth in human form, and as the Bible tells us, He was sinless. What we cannot fail to understand is that Adam was also sinless for a time, until Satan entered the scene.

So at the outset, when Adam was created, God said, "Let Us make man in Our image, according to Our likeness" (Gen. 1:26). Most theologians agree the scripture is referring to the outward appearance of God. This means that God is not fifty feet tall with wings. He has two eyes, ten fingers, and ten toes. But why would it be so important for God to tell us that man (including you) was created in His image? Well, it is because He wanted you to know that you are like Him. And since you are like Him, even beyond your outward appearance, it is important to understand the uniqueness of being created in His image.

No other living thing created by God (which means nothing in all of creation) is created in His image and likeness other than you and me. Isn't that absolutely amazing? Dogs and cats were not created in His image. Monkeys were not created in His image. Only we were. Only man reflects the outward appearance of God. It was critical that when Jesus came to earth as the Son of the living God, He looked like those with whom He dwelled.

Let's now take a look at 1 Thessalonians 5:23: "Now may the God of peace Himself sanctify you completely; and may your whole spirit, soul, and body be preserved blameless at the coming of our Lord Jesus Christ." This letter to the Thessalonians was written by Paul, inspired by God. In this passage the Bible shows us that Paul was praying for believers in Christ to be sanctified, that is, separated or set apart, to live a life free from sin. Read that scripture again and notice that Paul makes a distinction that sanctification should occur not just in body but in all three parts of man. My conclusion is that this articulates, or makes clear, that there are three unique areas that make up what I call the total composition of man. This is the triune you, the three parts that are affected by this world: spirit, soul, and body.

When I began this journey searching for how God cures, I had no real clue about these three parts of me. This is part of the grand delusion I spoke about in an earlier chapter. If Satan can keep people blinded to the realization of our three parts, then he can keep us from discovering how these parts, properly ordered, can lead to healing, being cured, and discovering why we were put here in the first place.

THE MIRROR OF THE WORD

Part of the reason Christians fail to understand these three unique parts of their composition is that many Christians (and I was one of them) go to church, sing some hymns, read a few scriptures, murmur a prayer, listen to the sermon, and then head right back to the life from which they came. You will not find out who you really are merely by attending church. The truth of who you are and how you are supposed to function is not found in just having a great prayer life. It is not found lying back on a therapist's couch. The place where you will find the truth, where you can stare into the mirror and see yourself for who you really are, is the Bible. The Scriptures, which are living and powerful, will reveal to you who you really are from the inside out and how you are intended to function.

> For the word of God is living and active and sharper than any two-edged sword, and piercing as far as the division of soul and spirit, of both joints and marrow, and able to judge the thoughts and intentions of the heart.
> —HEBREWS 4:12, NASB

Think about a time you had something in your eye. It irritated you so much that you ran to the mirror to find out what it was and to remove it. As a believer, that is what the Word of God does for you. It helps you identify what is wrong and helps you rid your life of it—but only if you listen to what God is telling you and act on it.

> But be doers of the word, and not hearers only, deceiving yourselves. For if anyone is a hearer of the word and not a doer, he is like a man observing his natural face in a mirror;

for he observes himself, goes away, and immediately forgets
what kind of man he was.

—JAMES 1:22–24

Now look at Hebrews 4:12 in the Amplified Bible:

For the word of God is living and active and full of power
[making it operative, energizing, and effective]. It is sharper
than any two-edged sword, penetrating as far as the divi-
sion of the soul and spirit [the completeness of a person],
and of both joints and marrow [the deepest parts of our
nature], exposing and judging the very thoughts and inten-
tions of the heart.

Notice that this amplified scripture indicates that each of us
has a spirit, a soul, and a body! It is God's Word that cuts deep
into your three parts, like a surgeon's scalpel, to show you who
you really are. The Word breaks you apart so you can be rightly
ordered again.

When we study the Scriptures, we find that God is triune,
which means that He is made up of three persons, three separate
entities, who are one—the Father, the Son, and the Spirit. While
we often address them uniquely and separately, together they represent God, the triune Godhead. In the same way, as we are created in their image and likeness, it reveals man as a triune being,
consisting of three parts that make up our total composition.

THE SOUL-LED LIFE

Let's take a trip to the beginning again. Genesis 2:7 reads, "And
the LORD God formed man of the dust of the ground, and
breathed into his nostrils the breath of life; and man became a
living being." Some other translations render the phrase *a living*

being as "a living soul" (e.g., KJV). Imagine God breathing life into man. His body was formed from clay, and man became flesh. This is what the Scriptures say. For the really deep thinkers, notice that Adam was not created in the garden. Genesis 2:8 says that God put him there after he was created.

So the soul was created, one part of the three that make up the whole man. I like what the late great Bible teacher and theologian Derek Prince had to say about the soul. His belief was that the soul is the ego of man: the will, the intellect, and the emotions.[2] My grandfather says that the soul is the seat of our affections. It drives our decisions in the natural—our wants, our opinions, and our feelings.

Just look around us in the media, in popular culture, and in the political realm, and consider what really drives humanity. I would say we are totally and completely soulish. Stop and consider what happened in the garden. Why did man sin? Simple. His ego was manipulated by Satan. The devil knew what buttons to push. He pushed the soul buttons. This suggests that Satan knew man's soulish character. Fascinating.

But here's the thing: man was not created to be soul led. In other words, man was not created to be led, be directed, or make decisions based upon his soul. Man was not created to make decisions or to lead his life based upon his wants. Please notice the lowercase *h*. Man was created to have a personal relationship with God, to have fellowship with God, and to be led by God's Spirit. Scripture suggests that there was a tight relationship between Adam and God.

> And they heard the sound of the LORD God walking in the garden in the cool of the day, and Adam and his wife hid themselves from the presence of the LORD God among the trees of the garden.
>
> —GENESIS 3:8

Some theologians believe that this verse suggests God and Adam used to hang out. I agree. If God was walking in the garden after sin, I think we can conclude that it was not God's first time walking in the garden. I think God cared about Adam and Eve enough to create them in His image, and therefore God likely visited them often. He walked in the garden amongst them. They could hear Him. They talked.

But you see, Adam and Eve's disobedience caused a tidal wave of problems, including what I believe was the first fracture in the total composition of man—soul decay, soul disruption. But it did not stop there. Each of the three parts of their composition was disrupted. Their bodies began to age, and sin caused them to be spiritually separated from God.

> And the LORD God commanded the man, saying, "Of every tree of the garden you may freely eat; but of the tree of the knowledge of good and evil you shall not eat, for in the day that you eat of it you shall surely die."
> —GENESIS 2:16–17

Die? But wait a minute—they didn't die! Did God change His mind? No. When God spoke those words, He was not referring to a physical death. God was not saying Adam was headed for the grave, at least not right away. Adam lived for more than nine hundred years. But physical death is what we think of when we read this passage. We read that man will surely die, and we take from that man is no longer immortal. It might be more than nine hundred years, but yes, man will surely die. But that is not what God was talking about! Most theologians believe that when God told Adam he would die, He was *really* talking about spiritual death.

Satan manipulated Adam, causing Adam to make a soul-led decision. Adam's decision was a direct violation of what God commanded him not to do. This disobedience forever changed the relationship Adam had with God and in turn defined our souls as having a predisposition for disobedience.

Look at this verse in Ephesians, the words of Paul inspired by the Spirit of God: "And you He made alive, who were dead in trespasses and sins, in which you once walked according to the course of this world, according to the prince of the power of the air [Satan], the spirit who now works in the sons of disobedience, among whom also we all once conducted ourselves in the lusts of our flesh, fulfilling the desires of the flesh and of the mind, and were by nature children of wrath, just as the others" (Eph. 2:1–3). That is the very definition of a soul-led life. It did not stop with just Adam and Eve. All of us were born outside of the garden. Since that very first rebellion in the soul against the will of God for mankind, every one of us has a propensity, an inclination or natural tendency, to follow our ego, our soul. Why? Because of sin, when we are born, we are dead in our spirits, completely subject to a soul-led life. We came out of the womb that way. We are three parts in one and yet completely soul led. And just like Adam and Eve, our bodies are subject to sickness and disease.

But know this: God has a plan. God wants you to be His. God wants you to be connected to Him. God offers you redemption and reconciliation and rebirth. Look at what James 4:4–5 says: "Do you not know that friendship with the world is enmity with God? Whoever therefore wants [or chooses] to be a friend of the world makes himself an enemy of God. Or do you think that the Scripture says in vain, 'The Spirit who dwells in us yearns jealously'?" I also like how the New American Standard Bible says that last part: "Or do you think that the Scripture speaks to no purpose: 'He jealously desires the Spirit which He has made to dwell in us'?" This means that God wants you.

So how does man get reconnected? How do you get connected to the God who yearns to dwell in you? It is quite simple—salvation.

> But God, being rich in mercy, because of His great love with which He loved us, even when we were dead in our transgressions, made us alive together with Christ.
> —EPHESIANS 2:4–5, NASB

It is at this critical time of salvation that man is finally reunited with God, that the spirit is regenerated, comes alive, is reborn. And this all starts with repentance.

> If anyone desires to come after Me, let him deny himself, and take up his cross, and follow Me. For whoever desires to save his life will lose it, but whoever loses his life for My sake will find it.
> —MATTHEW 16:24–25

Note that the word translated as "life" in Matthew 16:25 is the Greek word *psyche*, which also means "soul."[3]

AT THE CROSS

So where does death occur? This is not about the grave. This is about the cross! The cross is where we lay ourselves down. This is where we are reborn and our spirits regenerated. This is where our spirits take dominion over our souls.

This does not mean that we are robots. God gives us free will. But when the spirit is activated, we become connected to God's Spirit, and it is from His Spirit that man receives his marching orders in this life. We will spend the rest of our days at war with our souls, that is to say, we will have to fight to put God's will and wants for our lives ahead of our wants and our wills. This is a tension that we have to live with. Because of God's Word we know that our ways, wants, and wills are influenced by the world, and the world is influenced by Satan (Eph. 2:2–3).

As children of God, we can always remember the wisdom given to us by God through the prophet Isaiah: "For as the heavens are higher than the earth, so are My ways higher than your ways, and My thoughts than your thoughts" (Isa. 55:9).

When your soul becomes subject to your regenerated spirit, and as you seek God's will for your life through His Word, you find the life God intended for you. This is when you find your pathway to healing and to finally becoming cured as you eradicate what is inside you that leads to death and decay.

First Corinthians 6:17 reveals, "But he who is joined to the Lord is one spirit with Him." Is there any evidence of God's Spirit being sick or diseased? You won't find any. So if you are connected to God's Spirit, if you are one spirit with Him, which leads to life and happiness and health and wholeness, then what would your soul lead you to if your soul is connected to the world? You got it—it leads to the opposite of life and happiness and health and wholeness.

There are numerous places in the Bible where we find that it is through our spirits, not our souls or our bodies, that we have a close and intimate connection with God. (See, for example, Psalm 34:18; Proverbs 20:27; and Romans 8:14–15.) A close and intimate connection with God means walking in His grace, by His love, and toward the life He wants for us. And the life He wants for us does not involve sickness or disease.

When I was a boy, my father worked with the late Lester Sumrall. What a mighty man of God he was, a prayer warrior. He used to come to our home and eat dinner. My mother would make her amazing biscuits and gravy, and my father and Lester Sumrall would talk television business, ministry growth, and more. I would listen to them talk shop as I played with my action figures in an adjacent room. These are memories I will never forget. Even at age six, I remember the power and influence that such a mighty man of faith walked in. Lester Sumrall said that the spirit of man is connected to God, and the soul is connected to the world. How profound! So do you want to be connected to God or to the world?

If the spirit of man is getting insight, input, and direction from God's Spirit, the spirit is leading the soul, and the soul is leading the body, then that is the perfect setup for happiness, health, and wholeness. If that is the result of the three parts of you working in perfect alignment, then what is the end result of improper alignment? In other words, if the soul is leading the spirit (meaning the soul is in the driver's seat), what impact is it going to have on the spirit and the body since the soul is getting its marching orders from popular culture and whatever has a grip on your soul? By the way, I once heard it said that what you feed will grow. Consider this scripture: "For where your treasure is, there your heart will be also" (Matt. 6:21).

The news media, social media, the latest trends, fast cars, big houses, jewelry, sex, pornography, and countless other things can drive our soul-led lives. If your soul is leading in life, and your soul is getting its direction from the corrupt, toxic, depressed, distressed, sick, diseased, and addicted world, then where will you end up? Think about it.

Satan's goal is to dismantle you, one part (of three) at a time. The progression of erosion by sickness and disease will begin to manifest if and when the devil can move the three parts of you out of alignment through his schemes. We are about to dive deeper into this, as well as how to avoid it and how to repair and restore your inward and outward man.

Chapter 5

TAMING THE SOUL

I WOULD SAY THAT in my most sober moments, in the quiet times, in the dark of the night, if asked what I felt I was created to do, what I was meant to do, what I was put on this earth to do, it would be to sing. I dreamed as a child that I would sing. I believe I was born to do it. And yet it is only as I approach the midpoint of my life that I have finally discovered the voice God planted inside me.

The soul of man is a remarkable masterwork of a Creator that Himself is full of passion and full of emotions, the greatest of which is love. I am fully aware of this when I sing. I am without question one with the universe when I tilt the microphone and let loose. It is as though my insides resonate with the vibrations of the earth, the ebb and flow of God's creation, and I am floating with angels' wings. I am turned inward, tapping into the soul inside me, the soul God created with all of its passion, and giving the world what I have to offer.

Within your soul exists something capable of changing the world. Within your soul resides the power to shift thought, influence perceptions, and motivate the hearts of man toward the Cross of Jesus. It is for this reason that upon humanity's expulsion from the garden, they still had a remaining purpose on the planet and amongst the creation of God.

However, if Satan, the greatest liar of all liars, can influence you to believe that what you have in you, that gift, is yours to own, then he has accomplished his task of causing you to believe you actually have the power to control it. Satan's intent is to influence you to cover your gift, the one God planted inside you, and keep it from reaching the world.

SOUL POWER

When you understand the power of your soul, which I hope I have articulated well, you can then understand the stark reality that unless your soul is in subjection to your spirit, your soul's unbridled passion will be what ultimately wrecks your world. I have often wondered if at any moment along the musical journey of Elvis Presley, sometime before he influenced the world away from the Cross, the Cross was the true place his gift was designed to compel man. When we look at Elvis's life, a life celebrated because of his great success, we must pause to consider that it was also a life lived with great tragedy. Elvis Presley was depressed, medicated, obese, and uncontrolled. He lived a soul-led life.

Consider Michael Jackson. He was perhaps the greatest musical talent the world will ever know. Yet behind the splendor of such a great gift, his life was wrought with such pain, and it ended in such darkness, distress, sorrow, and loneliness.

Robin Williams made the world laugh. He hanged himself with his own belt.

Whitney Houston. She had a voice to stir angels, a voice that pushed past the church walls, but she was found dead in a tub, self-medicated and all alone.

I could fill the pages of this book with the stories of those whose lives were surrendered to the force of an enemy, whose gifts were captured by the devices of Satan and the luring appeal of what this world promises to offer. This world offers *nothing*. It offers nothing lasting, only temporary pleasures, in return for using us and leaving us spiritually bankrupt. Our time in the spotlight is brief, and we must recognize the brevity of our opportunity to find our gift and use it completely for the purpose of the Master. We were created to influence, and our gifts were to be used *in* this world, not to be lost to it.

Your soul is a power center, and getting your soul under control is going to be a daunting task. Believe me. It has led you for the better part of your life. It is not as easy as just saying, "Soul, submit to me!" If only it were so simple. Let's face it. Each morning you wake, you open your eyes, and your body screams for your morning routine. Mine includes coffee, freshly brewed, with two creams and half a sugar. Get up, get a shower, make yourself pretty, get in the car, and go to work—or some variation. Or perhaps it is all morning with the kids, readying the future minds of America for school while keeping the plates spinning in your family's world.

The soul is strong because we have been feeding it since birth. And what's more, everyone around us has fed it: parents, friends, family, teachers, and more. Our children cry, and we pacify them by meeting their emotional needs so we can finally find our own moments of peace. We feed them sugar, we put them in front of Saturday morning cartoons, and we find ways to give them happiness with toys, trinkets, and more. Within our entire circle the success of living is measured and governed by how we feel, by what we are fed. From our earliest years, our emotions are fed so that we determine health and well-being by how we feel.

As teenagers, the pursuit of gratification is insatiable. This voracious appetite to consume converts to how we measure up, whether or not we can compete and win, if we fit in, if we are liked, if we are considered popular, and none of it is geared toward caring for the spiritual part of our composition!

As we become adults, we are also led by our soulish nature. We pursue relationships based upon looks and how someone makes us feel. We search for features in a mate such as financial strength, what they have and have not. We rush into lifelong commitments, often driven by lust disguised as love, and say "I do" based upon short-term scorecards that show how the new mate measures up to old ones, and *maybe* we place weight on their spiritual beliefs or their relationship with the God we serve.

Are you seeing a pattern? So shouldn't we conclude that the soulish nature is synonymous with the emotional side of who we are? Yes. And the government, the educational system, corporations, and even the medical establishment firmly rely upon consumers making decisions *completely motivated by emotion.*

However, the reality is that most of us, if asked, would say we make decisions in a different way. We would say our decisions are based upon a logical approach to choices presented to us in a logical way. We would say we were presented these options, and we made the right choice, the smart choice, based upon the facts at our disposal. But this could not be further from the truth based upon scientific data and studies conducted by major universities. Such studies show that our decisions are significantly impacted, if not completely driven, by emotional responses to the options and alternatives presented.[1]

Antonio Damasio, a professor of neuroscience at the University of Southern California, wrote a book called *Descartes' Error*. He argues that one's emotions must be part of the process in order for a decision to be made. He goes on to say that our past experiences of similar situations where comparable decisions were being made factor in, and it will be emotional recall that will cause us to place value on the options later presented to us. He says our brain is designed this way.[2]

Advertising agencies know this, and they know it well. They sell to our emotions. They pull on our heartstrings, motivate us by our senses, and build dreamscapes to help us envision what life would be like if we could experience the benefits of a certain product. Media, entertainment, art, and popular culture push the felt-need buttons of our souls. And our souls, if not led by the Spirit of God, sit ready and willing to respond.

WHAT DOES IT TAKE TO CHANGE?

I can hear the words from long ago, "Young man, are you OK?" as if they were spoken aloud just now. I was lying on a shiny stainless steel table in a hospital operating room. It was cold and bright, and there was a flurry of activity as doctors, nurses, and technicians moved purposefully about the room. I was there because for the umpteenth time my heart was beating uncontrollably at two hundred and sixty-three beats per minute (BPM). I was twenty-seven years old and had been diagnosed with supraventricular tachycardia (SVT), a type of arrhythmia that springs from a malfunction of the heart's electrical activity.

My chest was pounding. I felt faint, short of breath, and dizzy. My heart disease was passed down to me from prior generations.

It had plagued me for years, even before we had a name for it and knew what to do. But starting in my early twenties the drill was to call 911, and when the paramedics arrived, they would inject me with Adenocard to slow down my heart rate. Then my heart would restart its electrical system at a more normal pace of sixty to eighty beats per minute. But this time the Adenocard didn't work. They tried it twice, but my heart kept racing. So, the paramedics drove me to the emergency room of the hospital and thankfully there were cardiologists available.

After I was transferred from the ambulance gurney to another gurney and wheeled to the operating room, one of the doctors who had been briefed on my condition came over to me. Leaning down close, the cardiologist asked, "Young man, are you OK?" It was not what he said that concerned me as much as the look in his eyes. He was scared.

I was scared too, even though I had carried this fracture in my genetic profile all of my life. In fact, I had "died" for a few seconds many times. And I admit that it was terrifying the first time they injected me with a heart-stopping drug and I did not know if I would ever wake up.

Remember that first time you lost your job or were broke? Or that first time you were hurt by a broken relationship or when you lost someone? Or that first time you were beaten as a child? Remember the first time something like that happened to you? It was scary at first, it was bad, and it was tough. Life has a way of kicking you in the teeth. It is so bad, and all you can see is struggle. You feel like you just can't win or get a break. You cannot get excited about anything. You do not want to be joyful or hopeful. In those times, Pastor Frank Santora says that even though they say, "When it rains, it pours," you need to choose to believe that "when it pours, God reigns."[3]

When the doctor asked me if I was OK, I was ready for the

worst. I had two thoughts hit me almost simultaneously: "I'm tired and don't want to do this anymore," and, "I'm at peace." If you have ever had your life pass before your eyes when faced with death, you know exactly what I was experiencing.

But here was the question as I lay there on that gurney: Would my last breath here on earth lead to me having an immediate encounter with my Creator, and would I be able to look Him in the eyes and tell Him I had lived the life I was meant to live?

I did not believe I was really going to die having not accomplished anything of importance. That would have been a cosmic joke, and I really did not believe that the God I had been taught loved me and loved the world would do that kind of thing. To that point, I really believe that people who take their own lives often do so because they think there isn't anything else and they have already lived their greatest moments. If only they would realize they were made to have a future and a hope. If only they could discover how to live lives ruled by their spirits, connected to the Spirit of God.

> For I know the thoughts that I think toward you, says the LORD, thoughts of peace and not of evil, to give you a future and a hope.
>
> —JEREMIAH 29:11

I survived supraventricular tachycardia. My eyes were opened by having such near-death experiences, and I wanted to know what God had for me since He was willing to heal me through the miraculous wonders of medicine and surgery. But I did not understand the power of my soul. I did not change my life, I did not change my thinking, and I continued to allow the world to influence all my doing. Within a decade I found myself battling an autoimmune condition that medicine described as incurable.

I realize now that I had been fighting Satan my whole life because I did not understand the destructive power of a soul-led life.

If the enemy can keep you from realizing the power inside of you, keep you from harnessing the power of your spirit connected to God's Spirit, and convince you to lean solely on the power of the soul, then you are in trouble! With the soul leading and the body in tow, you are subject to fractures in your total composition, and the natural progression from there is disease and death. By default, whatever gift is inside you will go to the grave with you, and the goal for you to live out your purpose and discover your destiny is lost.

We are not claiming sickness, but we are going to take the first step by *acknowledging it*. We have ignored it long enough. We are going to acknowledge that there are composition fractures, and that because we have allowed Satan to disorient us, disorganize us, and manipulate a misalignment, we have become unwell. The first step, even according to Alcoholics Anonymous, is to admit there is a problem. However, unlike AA, which supposes in its first step that one is "powerless" over addiction, we are instead declaring that *we have the power to change*. We are going to do something about what we have acknowledged.

THE PATH

Consider the lame man at the pool of Bethesda. Listen to his plight:

> Now there is in Jerusalem by the Sheep Gate a pool, which is called in Hebrew, Bethesda, having five porches. In these lay a great multitude of sick people, blind, lame, paralyzed, waiting for the moving of the water. For an angel went down at a certain time into the pool and stirred up the water; then whoever stepped in first, after the stirring of the water,

was made well of whatever disease he had. Now a certain man was there who had an infirmity thirty-eight years. When Jesus saw him lying there, and knew that he already had been in that condition a long time, He said to him, "Do you want to be made well?" The sick man answered Him, "Sir, I have no man to put me into the pool when the water is stirred up; but while I am coming, another steps down before me."

—JOHN 5:2–7

Are you kidding me? He was sick for thirty-eight years but did nothing! Couldn't he have rolled over to the edge of the pool at some point during those thirty-eight years? I'm serious! He acknowledges his sickness (step one), but then he does *nothing*, just depending on others to do it for him.

Not me and not you! You took step one by getting this book, and it is time for us to deal with your sickness!

We have the power to change! Why? Because we are not going to lean on our own understanding. We are going to lean on God, from whom we draw our power to conquer whatever plagues us.

Trust in the LORD with all your heart and do not lean on your own understanding. In all your ways acknowledge Him, and He will make your paths straight.

—PROVERBS 3:5–6, NASB

To be unwell is to say our path was not straight. Our path was bent, crooked. Satan influenced us to head down the wrong path, and he did it intentionally. There were signs along the way, but we ignored them. We trudged on. We therefore became sick. It's a natural progression. But we have been awakened to this reality, and it is not a reality that we have to live with or suffer through any longer. We have realized that we can take responsibility knowing we are in full and complete control to do something about it.

You see, God declared a different plan and a different path for you: "The mind of man plans his way, but the LORD directs his steps" (Prov. 16:9, NASB). Another translation says, "In their hearts humans plan their course, but the LORD establishes their steps" (Prov. 16:9, NIV). The grand delusion of Satan has been exposed. You now have an understanding of his plot, his scheme, his diabolical strategy to overtake you. However, Jesus came that you might have life and have it to the full!

> The thief comes only to steal and kill and destroy; I came
> that they may have life, and have it abundantly.
> —JOHN 10:10, NASB

God's great love covers a multitude of cracks in our fragile humanity, and God's great grace is always sufficient for us. He does not keep score. Our tragedies, our struggles, our stumbles, and our setbacks are nothing but a setup for God to show the world through our redemptive testimony that His redemptive power is able to do exceedingly, abundantly more than we could ever hope for or imagine (Eph. 3:20). And believe me, God is in the testimony business!

The enemy might be able to influence your soul, but he cannot touch your spirit. He cannot infect the regenerated spirit. He can only stir up what your soulish man is up for, causing your soulish pursuits to be dialed up so high that they push your spirit man way down. As a result, the only voice you hear is the voice of this world.

When we look at the stories of many people whose lives have been wrecked and brought to an early, empty end, we see that Satan worked against them to fracture and misalign their composition, and he started early.

When divorce fractured my home as a child, it was the first—and maybe the largest—diabolical rift in my life. From age six, I was living in a broken home. Everything stable and secure was ripped from beneath my feet, and I was facing a future without a father and with just my mother to cling to. She was more scared and lost than I was. I carried the weight of the look in my father's eyes when he told me, my brother, and my mother that it was over for a long time. The hurt and painful rejection grew in me, and without my father there to heal it and guide me, I became lost to the world.

I think that day a tiny crack formed in the triune part of me. My soul, with the raging emotions and the struggle to understand the world and circumstances I was facing, had no room left to hear the Spirit of God. And even though I grew up in a God-loving family, I never really understood that in times of such great distress, the very thing we must cling to is the saving grace of God. Prayer should have been our refuge. God's love should have been our strength, His Word a light unto our path (Ps. 18:1; 119:105). Instead, a young and suddenly single mother with a small, brown-haired, innocent boy turned to the world for answers.

FATHERS AND CHILDREN

Our earthly fathers are responsible for our genetic makeup, which encompasses who we are biologically, but even the greatest dads on earth are flawed to some degree because we all fall short of the grace of God. Our fathers are not perfect because their fathers before them were not perfect, and so we find ourselves in a cycle of fractured parenting. People today are dealing with so much generational garbage, it's insane! The sad part is many people do not understand where the root of their pain resides.

A stable, loving father is one who can provide wisdom, stability, and a feeling of security. This security provides the nurturing soil for the development of identity, and that identity, how we perceive ourselves, leads to our destiny.

I believe there is an instinctual desire in all children, no matter what part of the world they come from, to be loved, to have discipline, and to be parented. But without security and love, children grow up and evolve into broken adults. They live broken lives, and for the most part are bitter, resentful, and mad at the world. And often those children look for love in all the wrong places. Have you ever heard the song "To Be Loved" by Jackie Wilson? The world is crying out for love because it truly is the greatest feeling in the world. But that desire to be loved comes from God.

Whenever Jesus referred to God, for the most part He referred to Him as Father or Abba, which is a term similar to Daddy. Jesus, the Son of God, had a close and intimate relationship with God the Father, and once we accept Jesus Christ as our Savior, we are adopted into the family and can have the same intimate relationship. The Lord's Prayer begins with the words "Our Father in heaven" (Matt. 6:9). Have you ever considered the opening to that prayer? Jesus told us to refer to God as Father. He was responsible for our creation, and we are His children. First Corinthians 8:6 tells us, "Yet for us there is one God, the Father, from whom are all things and for whom we exist, and one Lord, Jesus Christ, through whom are all things and through whom we exist" (ESV).

God knew each one of us intimately since our conception. He planted and knitted us in the womb. He created us in a secret place. He loved us before anyone ever knew who we were. He knew our characteristics, the number of hairs on our head, and the number of our days. How incredible is that when you think about it deeply! Our earthly fathers have the potential for great parenting, but only our heavenly Father has a relationship with us that began on a cellular level. The level at which our heavenly Father knows us is incomparable since He molded and designed every aspect of our being. He is aware of every motivation, thought, and action. He knows us better than we know ourselves!

> Before I formed you in the womb I knew you, and before you were born I consecrated you; I appointed you a prophet to the nations.
>
> —JEREMIAH 1:5, ESV

God appointed us to be prophets to the nations before we were even born. We were established, preordained, and planned for this life. He designed every detail for our anointed lives. And if He designed us and appointed us, surely He will equip us with His grace and strengthen us for anything He has called us to do. Now that is what a father really is! A father creates, redeems, restores, establishes, and heals.

So where does the fracture Pastor Dickow speaks about fit into all of this? Hebrews 11:6 says, "And without faith it is impossible to please God, for he who comes to God must believe that He exists and that He is a rewarder of those who diligently seek Him" (MEV). God wants us to recognize Him as our Father, Creator, Defender, and Benefactor.

I shared a piece of my childhood with you so you could understand that everyone, no matter what walk of life they come from, is dealing with something. But God can rescue us from all our woes and usher in salvation. He can forgive all the iniquity present in our lives. God's healing, redemption, and restoration extend beyond building you back up as He seals you by His grace.

What does it mean to be sealed by God? Once you are reconciled to Him, you are sealed with the Holy Spirit (Eph. 1:13). When you are sealed by God, you have the promise of the Holy

Spirit. The Spirit of God is your security and your connection to the Father. That sounds very supernatural, doesn't it? And in fact, it *is* supernatural, because that is what God is. He is your supernatural Father, the part of you that empowers and guarantees your ability to conquer anything in your life. Sometimes you need to get out of your own way. Many times when you think you are broken, you are simply falling into place. You may come from a broken home or be in a failing marriage, but if you just step back and let God work in your life, He will restore any area of disconnect!

For generations the devil has been attacking the men in my family with disease and robbing them of life at an early age. The three generations before me—my father, my grandfather, and my great-grandfather—all passed before the age of sixty, and that was part of my impetus to begin this journey in the first place. What I discovered was the reality of the power of the soul, but even greater, the power of the spirit within us when connected to the Spirit of God. When this alignment occurs, the soul becomes a force for the kingdom. And when you are doing the work of the kingdom, your soul, led by your spirit, will have the kind of impact on the world that God wants most of all.

One day I got a phone call from one of my sons. He wanted to get together and talk about something on his mind. He wanted to talk to me and my wife together. Through FaceTime he showed me what his place was like. He was living in squalor in a run-down house with some people he did not know very well. I saw the pallet he was sleeping on in a corner, and the surrounding area was in a state of total disarray. As my son walked the phone through the different rooms, I saw a bedridden man about eighty years old. There was another man with dementia who was walking around in a trance like a zombie. I was shocked and appalled to see my son living in such conditions, and I had to ask myself what had gone wrong. He was only in his early twenties. He was miserable in his present circumstances, and his only means of income was washing dishes in a restaurant. I suggested starting over and managed to convince him to come home.

Now, keep in mind that I don't think I have been a horrible father. I didn't run around on my wife or abuse my kids, and I wasn't a drunk. I have always held a steady job and provided for my family. We had a nice home, I ran a business, and I was respected within the community. But the situation here begged the question, How did we get to this point? It tore the heart right out of me to see my child hurt, as I'm sure most of you protective parents have felt at some time or another. And when he requested to meet with me and his mother to tell us something, my mind raced due to his somber tone. What would he tell us? Maybe he was doing drugs or had been attacked. I went through every scenario in my mind. What could he tell us that required a serious sit-down?

What he told me turned out to be the biggest trigger to wreak havoc on my mind, body, and spirit. Though I was in pain because of my thirty-third nodule related to rheumatoid arthritis, and though I received the diagnosis of an autoimmune disease inflaming my body and killing me slowly, those things were not enough of a kick in the pants to wake me up from my slumber of denial. What finally woke me up to a need for change was my son telling me that he was not sure about God—if He was actually there.

That was a wake-up call for me. You see, I am part of the legacy of over five generations of men and women of faith, teachers and preachers of the gospel. I was running one of the largest faith-based agencies in the world to help spread and share the gospel of Jesus Christ around the globe. My son had been brought up to know the Word of God and had attended church all his life.

This was the ultimate screech on the record, even greater than being told that I had an incurable disease. In truth, I felt like I had failed my son. Was all that I poured into life and my family worth it if this is where we ended up? Where had I gone wrong? Had I invested so much into business, security, and things the world associated with success only to have failed at the most important things? Had I failed to live up to my responsibility as a father to instill faith in my children and teach them about God, the greatest treasure we will ever know? The crushing thought echoed in my head: a man can gain the entire world and lose his soul. The source was Matthew 16:26: "For what profit is it to a man if he gains the whole world, and loses his own soul? Or what will a man give in exchange for his soul?"

I reflected on my father, who had left this world with the figurative two bags of gold but realized too late he could not take it with him. Did I want to spend the rest of my days building bigger barns, buying nicer cars and fancy suits, and filling up our bank accounts but never truly feeding my spirit? Material things only bring momentary happiness meant to fill the vapid holes in our lives and temporarily assuage the wounds from our fractured state.

So when faced with the spiritual legacy (or lack thereof) I was leaving for my son, I took a long, deep look at myself in the mirror and acknowledged that I needed to survive to help save my son. And it hit me, almost as though God was nudging me in my spirit—what had my son seen or not seen in me that challenged his belief in God and the need for God in his life? I will tell you what he did not see. He did not see the joy of the Lord in me. He saw a man, his father, who was asleep in his spirit, leading a soul-led and soul-fed life. He saw a perpetuated lie of the devil as it pertains to what happiness really is in this world.

I faced the mirror and made my commitment: I will save

myself in order to save my son. I will show him that there is a supernatural God. I will show him there is something planted in me that God created, and I will find it and unleash it on the earth. I will show him that there is also something in him that is God-created, and with my help he is going to find it and unleash it too. I will show him he has a special, God-intended purpose.

> Beloved, I pray that you may prosper in all things and be in health, just as your soul prospers.
>
> —3 JOHN 1:2

Our soul will begin to prosper the way that God wishes it to at the moment we get serious about living the Spirit-led life. As we begin to live the Spirit-led life, our composition will align, and we will move into a state of homeostasis, fully balanced, and our body will heal itself, as it was designed to do. As we continue to walk in this aligned balance, we will reach the cure that God has in store for us, a state in which nothing is missing, nothing is broken, and everything is whole.

Chapter 6

WHO IS DRIVING?

I WILL NEVER FORGET learning to drive. It was later for me than most. The dysfunction of my childhood put me at a disadvantage, so I did not sit behind the wheel legally until I was nearly eighteen. I pretty much used my thumb to get around before then. Eventually I drove an old, used 1982 Chevy Chevette—the family jalopy my mother had passed down to my older brother and then to me. But I was ready. All I could think was, "This is mine, and I'm going to put the pedal to the metal." My emotions were running high. I had places to go and ladies to see, and of course I had to "get that paper." That's slang for "make money," according to my daughter Sydney.

As of this writing, Sydney just turned eighteen, and due to the natural and supernatural dysfunction from my childhood I inadvertently passed on, my daughter has only now started to drive. Like my father before me, I neglected my duty to usher her onto the highway at the correct time. Fractured lives lead to fractured lives.

In this chapter we will discuss how we must come to terms with patterns, habits, and ways of thinking that cause fractures and that cause us to perpetuate them. With God leading rather than our soul leading, we can repair fractures and not repeat them.

IN THE DRIVER'S SEAT

My family did not have much when I was growing up. After my parents split up, finances were always a struggle. My stepfather worked, but things were still tight. Child support was inconsistent, and so I worked too.

When I was sixteen, I came home one night and had a huge argument with my stepfather. It was the last straw. As a result of our disagreement, I packed up and left.

The only safe, stable place I could go to was my grandparents' house, so I loaded my car and drove to Virginia. The whole way I kept hoping I would not be pulled over for driving illegally without a license, but I was escaping to a refuge at my grandparents' home, no matter what. They were the calm and safe place in the storm. My mother was my world, but she could not protect me. I had experienced the last of my abuse from dysfunctional men led by soul-driven addictions.

I was finally safe and stable with my grandparents. But my grandfather could not afford to sustain me past putting a roof over my head and food on the table on a pastor's salary. As a teenager, I needed more than a place to stay and food, so I did what I needed to—I worked. But just getting by was not enough for me. I was *driven*. There was something inside me, deep in my

DNA, an expression of drive switched on in my genes, that had me working one job when I arrived, two jobs by the end of my junior year, and four jobs through most of my senior year.

I was pushing eighteen with dark hair and green eyes; they say that I looked like Speed Racer, but my Mach 5 was a Chevette with a stick shift. For those who do not know cars, imagine a Volkswagen Beetle and a Yugo had a baby; that's an '82 Chevette. Putting the pedal to the metal meant I was tearing up the asphalt at forty-five miles an hour, maybe fifty-five if I started at the top of a hill.

I lived in Alexandria, a city in northern Virginia right outside of Washington, DC. Having come from a little town called Sugar Hill, Georgia, where it was pretty easy for me to find my way around, I found myself a bit disoriented in a city full of turns and roads and yields and stops. All I had was a tattered map, which was also handed down through my family. Anyone older than thirty-five knows what I'm talking about. GPS was technology only found on *Star Trek*.

A map was the only way we found our way around back then unless we stopped and asked directions at a gas station along the way. You had to navigate yourself. You wrote down the address, you grabbed the map (and perhaps even stopped and asked for help along the way), and then you eventually arrived. And don't forget that to figure out how to get to where you were going you first had to find out where you were.

So let's travel back to the moment I screeched my Chevy around the corner after school, barreling toward the first of my three daily jobs. I only had fifteen minutes from when the school bell rang to the moment the restaurant supervisor clicked his pen and jotted me down as late. While my friends were headed to drama class and wrestling practice, both of which I would have loved to participate in, I was rushing to a restaurant at the mall, where I would bus tables for two to three hours. I would then sneak into the family restroom at the mall and sleep for half an hour before washing up in the sink and changing to nicer clothes. After that, two days a week I worked at a jewelry store, and three days a week I worked at the movie theater tearing tickets. I got off at 9:00 p.m., and I would meet up with my girlfriend. I had one hour to reconnect to something of substance in this life—emotion, intimacy, connection, communication.

I then drove to the parking lot of my next job. I parked in the back and climbed in the backseat of my car for another half hour of sleep. I then changed clothes in a restroom and raced to the back office of the Hilton, where I worked the night audit shift from 11:00 p.m. to 7:00 a.m. A buddy would cover the desk for me around 2:00 a.m. so I could sneak in another few hours of sleep in an unoccupied room. I would shower and dress, then report back to the desk by 5:00 a.m. At 7:00 a.m. I would race off to school, trying to make it to first period on time, but I was late several times a week. When the school day ended, I would race off to work again.

This was my world at seventeen—out of order, totally fractured, and a breeding ground for ruptures in my body, soul, and spirit.

Back to the first sentence of this chapter: I will never forget learning to drive. Yes, I learned to drive, but I was also *driven*. I wanted to succeed.

SELF-HELP

Drive is control. It is the power to jettison us from point A to point B. It is the push, the force, the inside fuel. Our emotions, our will, our wants, and our souls are all are part of drive. We come into this life, and circumstances teach us to drive. Our parents drive, but they are full of fractures of their own with their lives out of alignment, and they pass a lot of junk and bad habits down to us.

But it is really hard not to find yourself charged up about what a life led by the soul has to offer you. The famed Tony Robbins's teachings are all about awakening the giant on the inside of you. He is referring to you having the power to do anything and to a self-driven, self-willed, self-discovery process.[1] The Internet defines *self-help* this way: "self-guided improvement—economically, intellectually, or emotionally—often with a substantial psychological basis.... Self-help often utilizes publicly available information or support groups.... The connotations of the word...often apply particularly to education, business, psychology [the study of behavior and the mind—the soul] and psychotherapy."[2]

I am not an advocate of burning down the bridges to self-help tools and techniques. Nor am I, however, an advocate of starting there or ending there, or of traveling through life leaning on *self* to get down the road. The scripture from Proverbs bears repeating: "Trust in the LORD with all your heart and do not lean on your own understanding. In all your ways acknowledge Him, and He will make your paths straight" (Prov. 3:5–6, NASB).

If leaning on self-help was working for any of us, we would not be on this crooked path on the map today. Every day would not be such a struggle. But that is what happens when you start out on a crooked path. Traveling the not-straight path means it will take longer to get where you are going, it will keep you longer than you are willing to stay, it will take more from you than you are willing to give, and you will leave with less than you came there with.

We get up and go. We came out of the womb having to get up and go. No one handed us a GPS unit to navigate our way through life, so we do the best we can on our own. At seventeen I was no different. All I knew was that I had come from disadvantage, I was living in disadvantage, I was going to have to navigate disadvantage, and no one was going to help me other than me. With my '82 Chevette and four jobs, I did what I could on my own. I was self-helping.

Everyone interprets life just a little bit differently. People look at where someone starts in life, then judge them by who they end up being. So people look at the unstable, destructive, exhausting life that I led as a teenager. They see how bad it was. However, by all accounts, I am now a person of esteem that others in the body of Christ look up to. People are impressed by what I have accomplished in spite of the disadvantage I had to overcome. They judge my life by the outcome. However, they are making a determination by what they see on the outside when what happened on the inside is what matters most. And what was happening on my inside was establishing a pattern, built on fractures, that would cause a fractured life twenty years later—one of sickness and disease. This is the grand delusion that Satan perpetuates.

The world chooses to look at the end of a thing, and if the end of the matter matches the world's definition of what success should be, we stamp it with a seal of approval. We look on the outside. We see the soulish benefits of a soul-led life, and we determine whether a life is successful. This is what the self-help gurus tend to proclaim is a successful life—one that has all the appearance of success on the outside. They point to what we have built, how much money we have made, what degrees we have. None of it can be taken by anyone into eternity. We may be all put together on the outside, yet our marriages fail, our bodies become toxic, and we are sick, unhappy, and without peace.

And still we push ourselves. We push through, past the point of breakdown. In fact, pushing ourselves and pushing through, even when we do it to the point of sacrificing what really matters and at the expense of our health, is seen as admirable. And while it is important to have that kind of intestinal fortitude, the reality is that a soul-led life causes two things:

1. We miss tapping into God's on-board navigational system to help us keep from getting lost, to help us find our way if we do get lost, to help us avoid the potholes, and to get to where we are supposed to go.

2. The path we are on leads to sickness, disease, and a life cut short.

God's path for us is an easier one, and it was designed so that we would have good health.

> Take My yoke upon you and learn from Me, for I am gentle and lowly in heart, and you will find rest for your souls. For My yoke is easy and My burden is light.
> —MATTHEW 11:29–30

YOUR BODY IS A TEMPLE

When I was seventeen, I felt invincible. I was not thinking about what I was doing to my body, at least not the way God says I should have. And without His Spirit leading, I was not benefiting from God's GPS.

Our bodies are temples, and we will start here:

> Do you not know that you are the temple of God and that the Spirit of God dwells in you? If anyone defiles the temple of God, God will destroy him. For the temple of God is holy, which temple you are.
> —1 CORINTHIANS 3:16–17

I'm going to linger for a minute and use my Chevette as an example. It got me to where I needed to go, but I destroyed it in the process. I was so busy abusing it to get me from here to there that I forgot to change the oil. I shot out the engine. Though I tried to fix it up, it was in the end a jalopy, dead on the side of the road. I ultimately sold it to a guy at a junkyard who chopped it up for parts. So much for self-helping!

But here's a thought. God does not make Chevettes. God makes Ferraris, even if you feel as if you have turned into a jalopy, dead on the side of the road. Let me remind you what the Word says:

> I will praise You, for I am fearfully and wonderfully made; marvelous are Your works, and that my soul knows very well.
>
> —Psalm 139:14

> Then all your people will be righteous and they will possess the land forever. They are the shoot I have planted, the work of my hands, for the display of my splendor.
>
> —Isaiah 60:21, NIV

> For we are God's masterpiece. He has created us anew in Christ Jesus, so we can do the good things he planned for us long ago.
>
> —Ephesians 2:10, NLT

You are a Ferrari, not a Chevette. You might feel like a Chevette, but God is going to cure that thinking. You are a Ferrari because God built you. And He built you to be a temple. A temple for what? Read 1 Corinthians 6:19: "Do you not know that your bodies are temples of the Holy Spirit, who is in you, whom you have received from God? You are not your own" (NIV). It does not say that your body is a temple of the soul. I cannot find anything in Scripture to support that statement. You can only find that adage with new-age thinkers. They postulate that in fact the spirit and the soul are one. They lean on the soul of man, and their doctrine, the doctrine of the world, says that we should rely upon it, tune it up, feed it, and send it out to battle. But the Scriptures state clearly that your body is the temple of His *Spirit*.

Your body is a temple. God made it. He has purpose for it. And He bought and paid for it through His Son.

> For you were bought at a price; therefore glorify God in your body and in your spirit, which are God's.
> —1 CORINTHIANS 6:20

A Ferrari is high tech. It is computer run and has an onboard navigation system. You can put the pedal to the metal and push that thing from zero to sixty in less than three seconds. When it comes to finding your way, you can use the navigation system in that supreme machine, and you never get lost. There's no pulling over to the side of the road and asking for directions. There's no unfolding the map on the hood and trying to find where you are and determine the best route to get from A to B. You're driving a Ferrari!

When we take time to slow down and look at the map of our life, it is usually only when we are lost. We have been treating our life like the Chevette, perhaps because we forgot that God made us a Ferrari. We have been going at it on our own. I like what Pastor Frank Santora told me when we were discussing this book and the Chevette-versus-the-Ferrari analogy. He said, "It's like we have this Ferrari that has all this power and can take us anywhere we want to go, and we keep getting lost behind the wheel because we keep trying to find our way on our own. The designer made the machine with a body that has such power and ability, and he put behind the wheel man, able to hit zero to sixty in three seconds, and also gave him access to intelligence to drive with precision, to reach the right destination, safely, peacefully, every time we get behind the wheel. But instead of tapping into it, God's Spirit, we go at it alone."[3]

LETTING GOD LEAD

By the last semester of my senior year, I was a wreck. I was tired and burnt out, my grades were terrible, and my crazy schedule was no longer sustainable. I walked into my grandfather's room one day and announced, "I can't do it anymore." After a long talk with my grandfather, I weighed all my options and decided the system was not for me. I dropped out of school, packed up, moved out, got my GED, and went into the world in full control of myself. Or so I thought.

We need to use God's Word instead of our finger to determine where we are on life's map. We need to use God's Word to determine if our life is in line with the destination He planned for us. When we look into the mirror of God's Word, it is apparent that with all of our confusion, frustration, depression, financial woes, relationship issues, addictions, health challenges, and the fact that we are worn slap out (as my grandmother used to say), God is not leading our lives.

> Do not merely listen to the word, and so deceive yourselves. Do what it says. Anyone who listens to the word but does not do what it says is like someone who looks at his face in a mirror and, after looking at himself, goes away and immediately forgets what he looks like. But whoever looks intently into the perfect law that gives freedom, and continues in it—not forgetting what they have heard, but doing it—they will be blessed in what they do.
>
> —JAMES 1:22–25, NIV

I call God's Word a mirror not simply because James refers to it as one but because when we look into a mirror, it gives us an honest, emotionless, factual representation of what the world sees. I'm not talking about one of those funny mirrors from the old circus days that warped your face or made a skinny person big and a big person small. I do like the funhouse mirror. I keep one in my production studio green room. It helps encourage me before I step in front of the camera and have ten pounds added onto me. I am in the television business, and I work with ministries and humanitarian organizations all over the world. We produce a lot of television programs out of our studios near Atlanta. My production and television career began with me working alongside my father with everyone from Benny Hinn to Joel Osteen. In the early days of learning television production, I remember thinking, "Wow, cameras really make us look good." Camera technology then was such that with the right lighting, lenses, makeup, and focus you could make anyone look like a Hollywood actor.

Today we have HD, and soon we will be shooting everything on 4K and higher. Because of their power, these cameras show everything, every one of our flaws. It is almost as though technology has downgraded us, because now everything looks so real to life, with no filter. Though we may say we want authenticity, none of us really want the world to see us as we really are. We like the filtered version. We like to wear our masks.

Negative Thoughts

During my journey to finding how God cures, I had the privilege of having Dr. Caroline Leaf, who has a PhD in communication pathology, as my guest on *IonONE* at our Legacy Worldwide television studios. During our time together, we produced two television programs: one on her book *Switch On Your Brain* and the other on her book *Think and Eat Yourself Smart*. Dr. Leaf helped me understand the immense power of our brains. During our two hours on camera together, I realized how many of my thoughts might need sorting out. I suspected I was dealing with toxic thinking. In my effort to stop living a soul-led life and allow God's Spirit to lead my spirit and my spirit to lead my soul so that my body would become healed, whole, and cured, Dr. Leaf helped me see very clearly.

Dr. Leaf shared that over 75 percent of the sickness we deal with is directly connected to our thought life. In other words, the stuff we think about directly impacts us emotionally and in a physical way in our bodies. She told me the world is facing an epidemic of toxic emotions. Dr. Leaf revealed that most people think thirty thousand to sixty thousand thoughts a day. She provided a theory that if our thought life is without control, then we set ourselves up to develop a whole host of sicknesses. We hang on to toxic stuff we should be releasing, such as grudges and resentment, thereby building barriers to getting well. Unforgiveness, as described by Dr. Leaf, is like toxic waste in our brain, and when it is not dealt with, it can cause diabetes, cancer, asthma, skin problems, allergies, and more.[4]

Dr. Leaf motivated me! Yet it was not the first time this revelation was introduced to me. Creflo Dollar taught me the power of my thought life—that my thoughts would drive my speaking; my speaking, my actions; and my actions, my outcome. My thoughts were a mess; therefore, my actions were a mess; therefore, my life was a mess. Pastor Gregory Dickow walked me through several lessons about how God changes us from the inside out and that the battlefield was always in my mind. Derek Grier showed me that healing and wholeness was found in walking daily with God in His Word.

But I was ready this time. Dr. Leaf's explanation of how my brain worked came when I was finished trying to do it on my own. I decided to see a Christian therapist. For the record, there is nothing wrong with seeing a professional with a thorough understanding of how the brain works and how we process emotions. There is nothing wrong with seeking professional assistance from an expert in the area of mental health. So I decided to visit a therapist suggested by Dr. Leaf. After our program wrapped, I called a local expert and set up some talk time to start to detox my thinking. Living a Spirit-led life leads to your thought life being led by God. God wants to dispel toxic thinking and help us learn to control our emotions so our emotions do not control us.

Creflo Dollar shared with me that emotions are designed to move us in a certain direction. There are so many negative emotions pushing and pulling at us. Almost all of them are the result of speaking negative words that are in opposition to God's Word. During my time with him, we talked about his own journey. He was diagnosed with a medical issue when Satan attempted to attack him in his thought life. A spirit of fear tried to creep in. He shared that when negative emotions come at us, we have to decide whose words we will give attention to. Will we give attention to God's Word, or will we focus on the lies of the enemy? If we allow Satan's word to reign, we will become prone to negative thoughts, which will lead to emotions that are against God's Word.

These powerful emotions can move us in a certain direction, but they need not steer our life. Our emotions cannot be what determine the direction we go! Creflo Dollar showed me that when we have negative thoughts, we must submit them to what the Word of God says about our circumstances. Getting my thoughts to line up with what God's Word says about me, my finances, my relationships, and my health will keep negative emotions from erupting and wrecking my life. And as Dr. Leaf showed me, negative emotions convert to a toxicity that can harmfully impact the body at a cellular level. Negative thinking equals negative emotions equals flipping a switch for sickness and disease expression in your genes.

This is not a hypothesis or a theory. This is God's Word, now proven by the revelation of epigenetics. God's Word and the leading of His Spirit helped me discover the power of positive emotions, emotions that trigger positive things. Positive emotions are healing. Positive emotions drive out toxicity. Leaning in and dwelling on what God's Word says leads to positive emotions and to cellular healing—the way God cures.

Detox Your Thinking

> My son, give attention to my words; incline your ear to my sayings. Do not let them depart from your sight; keep them in the midst of your heart. For they are life to those who find them and health to all their body. Watch over your heart with all diligence, for from it flow the springs of life.
> —Proverbs 4:20–23, NASB

Changing your thinking, moving away from a soul-led life and toward a Spirit-led life, is essential as you begin detoxing your thinking. This requires you to be in control of your thought life, and you must also look into the mirror of God's Word. This process starts with prayer. Just talk to God like He is your Father—the One who does not judge you, loves you unconditionally, is always there to listen to you, and is always ready to help.

God is our refuge and strength, a very present help in trouble.

—Psalm 46:1

If you then…know how to give good gifts to your children, how much more will your Father who is in heaven give good things to those who ask Him!

—Matthew 7:11

But you need to do more than just talk to God. You need to allow God to speak to you. And one of the ways God speaks to you, revealing what you need to see about yourself, others, life, decisions, and so much more, is through His Word, the Bible. Many people look at the Bible as an out-of-date history book that is no longer relevant. Just the opposite. God's Word is for today.

The grass withers, the flower fades, but the word of our God stands forever.

—Isaiah 40:8

For as the rain and the snow come down from heaven, and do not return there without watering the earth and making it bear and sprout, and furnishing seed to the sower and bread to the eater; so will My word be which goes forth from My mouth; it will not return to Me empty, without accomplishing what I desire, and without succeeding in the matter for which I sent it.

—Isaiah 55:10–11, NASB

Remember your leaders, who spoke the word of God to you. Consider the outcome of their way of life and imitate their faith. Jesus Christ is the same yesterday and today and forever. Do not be carried away by all kinds of strange teachings. It is good for our hearts to be strengthened by grace.

—Hebrews 13:7–9, NIV

Looking in the mirror of God's Word cannot be a casual glance. You must get up close to it. You need to get into the Word with the expectation that the Word will tell you where you are on the map. The Word will tell you how you are doing. The Word will give you an accurate depiction of how you *really* look and then guide you about what to do and how to do it by aligning your thinking with the Word.

But this is where things can break down and why so many in the body of Christ are still struggling and lost. We go to church. We pray. We tithe. We give to ministries. We read God's Word. We look into the mirror. We get conviction because we are suddenly exposed to a contradiction to our soul-led journey, but then we get up the next day and keep going on our soul-led course. So things never change. Some of us feel entangled. The web is so thick. The weeds are so high. The ties that bind are so strong.

We need the sharpest blade on earth to cut us out! Or maybe we need a sword—a double-edged one:

> For the word of God is living and powerful, and sharper than any two-edged sword, piercing even to the division of soul and spirit, and of joints and marrow, and is a discerner of the thoughts and intents of the heart.
>
> —HEBREWS 4:12

When I read God's Word, leaned on it, and went to it for answers even when my emotions led me in a different direction, the Word soon began to loosen the hold my soul had on my spirit. As God's Word cuts, we will see ourselves and our circumstances for what they really are. We will learn to master our emotions by mastering our thinking. As our thinking lines up with God's thinking, things change. It's that simple.

God's Word helped me see I was entangled. I had been living for so long driven by my soul that my entire thinking system was entangled. And my life was entangled because my thinking was entangled. I was dealing with some serious stuff beneath the surface: abuse as a child, betrayal, fear, anger, unforgiveness.

Through walking in God's Word, my responses to situations changed. I found myself feeling as though I was traveling lighter and breathing easier. I woke in the morning less stressed and less strained. It seemed as though my thinking was clearer.

I discovered it was not up to me to find my way on my own. I discovered that God made me a Ferrari, not a Chevette. As I began to see my life through God's Word, I found that God's Spirit was leading my spirit, and as a result I began to see myself as important and valuable. I finally realized how my actions, decisions, and lifestyle had led to the abuse of my body, which was wrecking me from the inside out. I ultimately took an inventory of my circumstances and asked God where *He* wanted me to be. I began to seek God about my situations, navigating them by His Word and with His Spirit leading my spirit, as opposed to allowing my will, my wants, and my emotions to guide me.

> Walk by the Spirit, and you will not carry out the desire of the flesh.
>
> —GALATIANS 5:16, NASB

As God's Word begins to divide our soul from our spirit and we begin to walk by the Spirit and not by the flesh, we find that our spirit begins to lead and God's Spirit and His Word become the GPS system that guides our life into better overall health. This is the way God cures.

Chapter 7

THE BODY

I HAVE BEEN ASKED a few times if I could give the elevator speech (what you could say just in the time it takes to ride the elevator with someone) on God cures. My elevator speech goes something like this:

God made you for a purpose. He put you on earth to do something big, great, and unto Him for His glory; to exalt and magnify His love and grace; and to demonstrate His power to mankind! Satan knows this, and from the moment you came out of the womb, he was on a mission to keep you from your destiny. How does he do this? He nudges you along the way to move you out of alignment. If he can move you out of alignment and keep you out of alignment, then that will affect your total, triune composition. There is a grand delusion at play. Satan has discovered that if you become sick, then sickness will lead to disease, and disease, to death. You will end this life not knowing who you are, having failed to discover what God created you to be, and the purpose, the gift, He planted in you will be taken to the grave.

I have discovered what makes man sick. It is misalignment. Misalignment is like your car. You're driving down the road, but it gets out of alignment and the wheels begin to shimmy and shake. Untreated, your car breaks down, and you're stuck on the side of the road. This is the enemy's strategy. This is his way to entrap you. The longer you run out of alignment, the longer you ignore the way your body is designed to operate, the more your body, soul, and spirit veer off the road and to a natural progression toward the grave. Misalignment is when the soul leads and the spirit is depleted and silenced. The impact of a soul-led life disables the body. The disabled body keeps your gift buried and your purpose unfulfilled.

In the last few chapters, we have discovered what a soul-led life means. We have discovered how to untangle the spirit from the soul and move into a place where our spirit is leading. This is how we move into homeostasis, which by definition is "a state of equilibrium (balance) of the interdependent elements (parts) of the body (our total self)."

Misalignment is what messes up the body's natural, God-designed function. When the body moves out of the order God designed for it, it gets on that slippery downward slope to declined health and more.

When you really think about it, Satan doesn't even have to work that hard to move us out of alignment. As indicated in previous chapters, we came out of the womb destined for trouble. (See Psalm 51:5; Romans 5:12; and Ephesians 2:3.) All the devil has to do is nudge us along the way, and we move into full-fledged misalignment.

When I discovered what was going on in my body was really a master strategy of Satan to kill what God put in me for the world to see, it really got me motivated. Looking back, I can see the devil's handiwork to stop me at every turn and impede me at every step in my acceleration toward my destiny. It isn't hard for Satan to keep our spirits silenced and our souls in the lead. Our souls are hungry. They need to be fed to satisfy their emotional vacancies. We need to be happy. We need to feel wanted. We need to be liked. We need to have control. We want everything to be easy. All Satan has to do is help us medicate ourselves with things that temporarily satisfy our dysfunctions, which is to say, help us temporarily fill the holes of despair rather than finding eternal gratification.

EMBRACE THE STRUGGLE

The enemy says, "Do it now. Get it fast. It'll be easy. It'll be quick. You won't have to work so hard. Take the easy way out." But I like what M. Scott Peck said in his book *The Road Less Traveled*: "To live wisely, we must daily delay gratification."[1] When we look at the life of Jesus and the lives of the apostles, we see successful people who know that struggle is resistance exercise for building our muscles of faith. It is what James talked about in the Bible:

> Consider it pure joy, my brothers and sisters, whenever you face trials of many kinds, because you know that the testing of your faith produces perseverance. Let perseverance finish its work so that you may be mature and complete, not lacking anything.
>
> —JAMES 1:2–4, NIV

James is saying we should embrace the struggle. Embrace the testimony God has written for your life. God is bringing you to a place of transcendence over the prince of the power of the air. You are rising above the devil. And you will be able to look back and see that this life has nothing you want to hold on to. Jesus asked the question, "What good is it for someone to gain the whole world, yet forfeit their soul?" (Mark 8:36, NIV). That verse reminds me of the final moments of my father's life when he said, "I have two bags of gold, and I can take nothing with me."

My friend Bishop Derek Grier said, "The fact you are in the battle only means you have something worth fighting for!"[2] You have a lot to fight for.

The body is an amazing machine. God told us that our body is a dwelling place of His Spirit. He bought us with a price; our body is not our own. But why has sickness come to rest on our doorstep? Can we really get into alignment and get out of where we are and on the track to becoming healthy? Is it all about delaying our gratifications, praying hard, reading the Word, and yielding to the leading of God's Spirit so the rest takes care of itself?

All of the above is important. Without these basic fundamentals, we might get healed, but we will end up sick all over again. Because most of us are so out of whack in the areas of our emotions and thinking, and because our spirits are so depleted, the process to get healthy and whole can be nearly impossible. We can eat right and exercise, yet anything we do in the physical can be completely derailed by our out-of-order thoughts and feelings and our spiritual disorder.

My attending physician, Dr. Joe Clarino, told me, "Before we can attack the physiology, we have to first deal with the psychology."[3] Since you understand the soul and spirit parts of the triune you, you can understand what Dr. Clarino meant. Once you start the process of alignment and then getting your body repaired, working with God to eradicate sickness and disease

becomes easier. He cures, and you become the properly functioning, rightly aligned you, and then, and only then, can you do
what my friend Joel Osteen says: "Live your best life now."

I met Joel in August 2004. My father worked with Joel to build
a television media distribution architecture for his media ministry that would help him reach millions of people worldwide
and outpace the news in terms of popularity in many major US
markets. When I met Joel, I told my father that I believed Joel
would reach people in a way that modern Christianity had never
done before. Having come from the infomercial industry as a
guy who had to figure out how to convince people to buy products, I specialized in touching felt needs. I told my dad, "Joel
touches felt needs like nothing I've ever seen. He presents the
good news of the gospel, and in a way in which someone in the
dark night of the soul can understand."

My father couldn't make it to Joel's first Night of Hope conference, which was being held at Philips Arena in Atlanta. He
asked if I would go for him to represent the agency. I said, "OK,
but Dad, I may not be able to stay." What I was telling my father
was that I did not mind going to represent the family, meet Joel,
and maybe shake his hand and such, but I was not about to sit
on the pew at some preacher's event. Keep in mind that at this
time in my life, my soul was still very much in the driver's seat.
I lived in Atlanta at the time, so I was only a forty-five-minute
drive away; I could go to the arena, take care of business, and be
back home by 8:30.

I asked my wife to join me, and we headed out to arrive at the
arena a few hours before the conference began to avoid traffic.
Dad told me that if I arrived early I could connect with the
people I needed to see, meet Joel, and then get a good seat. But
of course I had no intention of getting a good seat.

When we arrived at the arena, I was shocked; we couldn't find parking. We had to park in a parking deck at another building altogether and walk half a mile to the arena. I was mad, and my emotions were in full-swing. I actually cursed on the way over. (My wife reminded me of that.)

The place was packed. It was still hours before the event started, and there were several thousand already standing in line waiting to get in. We called on the chief of staff of the ministry, who greeted us and brought us inside. I remember making our way past the immense crowd, with some people wondering who we were—me in my perfectly fit Hugo Boss suit, Bruno Magli shoes, and Vacheron Constantin watch. The high school dropout from a broken home had come a long way. What they didn't know was that I was completely spiritually deplete. My soul was raging. And what I didn't know was I was sick inside at the cellular level. But at that moment, I was the man, and I was going to meet the man. I had the whole world fooled.

The arena filled to overflowing. My wife, Nathalie, and I exchanged hellos with the necessary people. Cindy Cruse Ratcliff and Israel Houghton were practicing "I Am a Friend of God," and it was time for us to roll. I called my dad and gave him a report. He said, "Enjoy the show, son," and I made my way toward the back door, leaving our front row seats unoccupied. I told Nathalie, "Let's go while we still can." We walked back to the parking deck and my waiting Mercedes.

And there I stood, staring in disbelief. My car was waiting, flat tire and all. I was mad as mad could get. My soul was raging.

Nathalie put her hand gently on my shoulder and said, "Perhaps God wants us to stay." (Thank God for our wives, gentlemen.) Now, don't mistake me. I am not suggesting God gave an angel a switchblade to puncture my tires so I would have to endure a "Night of Hope." So I'll let the Word say it: "But as for you, you meant evil against me; but God meant it for good" (Gen. 50:20).

I have no doubt that Satan rolled up into that parking deck and jacked my tire. And when I saw that tire, I was ready to curse. The devil thought he would cause me to see this setback as failure. My soul was so amped up and glued to the world that all the devil had to do was nudge me with my emotions, and my emotions did the rest. I sincerely believe Satan's goal was to distract me, to make me believe that this is how things go when you try to do something good for Jesus. I was standing in a hot parking deck staring at a flat tire and seething while thousands of people sat across the street to hear about hope.

But then there's God. And in that moment, He had a plan. My wife, in a sweet and encouraging voice, said, "I can call the roadside assistance. It will take twenty minutes for them to get here, maybe longer with all the traffic. Let's go inside. We have a front-row seat to hear Joel. We have to wait anyway. Let's at least wait inside in a comfortable seat, in air-conditioning, and in thirty minutes or so we'll be on our way." It seemed logical, and I conceded.

And then my life was moved toward change. My car being disabled was not God cursing me, just like your body being disabled is not God cursing you. God doesn't operate that way, in my opinion. I do not believe God flattened my tire that day, but I do believe He used that flat to get me to look at things differently, to pause and take inventory, to slow down long enough to see things the way *He* sees them. And He is going to use your health challenge the very same way.

If I had not sat in that arena that night, I would not have reconnected to the truth that I am a friend of God and that His grace, love, and power are able to do what my soul-led life could never do.

PAY ATTENTION TO THE WARNING

We cannot ignore how our bodies function and how they react to the years of a soul-led life. The flat, or that doctor's warning, may be God's opportunity to speak to us during a pause in the timeline of our life. God used that flat to pause me long enough to get some information that started me on my journey of discovery. And God is using what is going on in your body the same way. Your body has gotten sick by your own doing, along with the gleeful nudging by Satan, but God is going to use what the enemy meant for your harm for His good.

God will use a pause to cause us to be open to His Spirit's leading. God wants to cure you by eradicating bad thinking. God wants to cure you by eradicating your instinct to allow the words that come out of your mouth to direct your atmosphere and your emotions to drive you. God wants you to cling to His Word and allow His Spirit to take residence inside you, lead you, and move you in His direction on the path to wholeness. God is able to do exceedingly, abundantly, more than you could imagine was possible.

> But Jesus looked at them and said to them, "With men this is impossible, but with God all things are possible."
> —MATTHEW 19:26

You picked up this book. Perhaps this pause was God's way to introduce something new to the equation, just as He did for me in that parking deck. Now our job is to look deeply. Listen. Learn. Apply the information, the strategy, the revelation God has introduced to our situation.

The body is designed (created by God) to heal itself. For example, when we are wounded, blood rushes to the injured area, and the process of healing begins.[4] Blood rushing to an area of the body is known as inflammation. Inflammation, in its basic form, is healthy.[5] It is how God made the body. Inflammation is the first response to injury, and it is necessary for the process of healing to begin. Acute, prolonged inflammation, however, is the basis for nearly all disease.[6]

Did you get that? Inflammation is natural; it is good. But too much inflammation is bad. Inflammation at the right level heals; inflammation at the wrong level kills.[7]

The doctors tell me that my flat tire started with something going on in my gut. My condition is referred to as autoimmune, and it is there because of stress, poor diet, antibiotics, pain-killers, sugar, alcohol, no exercise, some genetic issues, and per-haps all those shots I received when I took humanitarian trips to other countries. I have what is called intestinal permeability, or leaky gut.

In the simplest of terms, my body breaks down food in my digestive tract, my gut. The gut has a lining that looks like cheesecloth with tiny little holes. These microscopic holes are there intentionally by God's design. They allow nutrients and minerals to travel into the body and bloodstream. When our gut is damaged, these holes become damaged and larger, allowing larger proteins and fragments to pass through along with the good stuff. These particles enter the bloodstream, and as a result the immune system goes haywire. This activity causes prolonged and painful inflammation. In other words, my immune system, which was designed to fight infection, turned on my body. Inflammation then became common, sustained, ongoing, and never yielding.

When I started doing research to find a solution, I discovered a lot about food and the marketing of food. You know all the food on the inside ring at the supermarket? Don't even buy it! Most of the food on the outer rim of the store is pretty good, especially the fresh veggies. And most of the rest of the foods are laden with chemicals we can't pronounce. You can read a list of all the sweeteners, sugars, and genetically modified foods on the box. These things are killing us by breaking down our organs.[8] These products make us feel good, but they are slowly bleeding us of our lives.

Most people struggle with inflammation, but they just don't know it. In nearly every known disease, including heart disease, diabetes, and arthritis, a baseline contributor is inflammation.[9] I am not talking about good inflammation, like when we get a scratch and the body sends inflammation to the cells around it to heal it. I am talking about prolonged, acute inflammation that stays in your system, leading to a whole host of diseases. A lot of people don't know about this. They walk around with digestive issues, bloated and lethargic. They cannot sleep and have brain fog.

We can make a list of all the issues we invite into our lives because of inflammation, which has been triggered by something aggravating the natural harmony and function of our bodies, spirits, and souls. We have to take inventory of ourselves. I am beginning to make a list. I am setting goals not about where I want to be in five years but instead about how to achieve harmony and balance in my life, how I want to change in my thinking, my will, and my emotions. My goals are about how to subtract things I know have fractured my total composition.

The goal of this journey is to bring balance. In bringing balance, we can prove the theory that the body will heal itself. I am tackling the war on my body differently. I have gotten my soul under control; my spirit is leading. And I have brought a team of health experts onto the field of battle with me.

Dr. Joe Clarino is one of the best all-natural wellness practitioners in the country. He is my attending physician, a man of God, a whiz on how the body works, a chiropractor, and an expert in cellular healing.

K. C. Craichy is my lead nutritional advisor. K. C. is the author of the best-selling books *Super Health—Seven Golden Keys to Unlock Lifelong Vitality* and *The Super Health Diet: The Last Diet You Will Ever Need!* K. C. is a sought-after speaker on the topics of nutrition, faith, life change, and overcoming obstacles. His approach with me, working with Dr. Clarino, has been a natural one to health and healing and encompasses lifestyle, nutrition, and fitness.

And that is where my dear friend and wellness colleague Dr. Joseph Christiano comes in. Dr. Christiano, a naturopathic doctor and certified nutrition consultant, is a recognized authority on redesigning the body. He is a health and fitness expert and the author of several best-selling books, such as *Bloodtypes, Bodytypes and You*. His exercise programs and lifestyle coaching have been embraced by celebrities such as Sylvester Stallone and women competing in the Miss America and Miss USA pageants.

I have learned so much about the body on this journey. During the balance of the book, I want to expose you to the truths I have come to know and how I have applied them to my lifestyle, each and every one having a remarkable impact on my physical healing. I believe they have helped me eradicate junk from my body that otherwise would keep me ill, diseased, and ultimately take my life.

The devil is a liar. And God is always on time when we are ready to receive what He has for us. He has your cure in mind.

There is a God in heaven who reveals mysteries.
—DANIEL 2:28, ESV

He reveals mysteries from the darkness and brings the deep
darkness into light.

—Job 12:22, nasb

Call to Me, and I will answer you, and show you great and
mighty things, which you do not know.

—Jeremiah 33:3

Sleep

Imagine if I told you that sleep was something that God gave
man to heal his body. I used to run from a good night's sleep. I
had so much going on in my life, so much to do and not enough
time to do it in, I had fallen into a pattern of sleeping less than
five hours a night. But as I have learned through the expertise of
my health and wellness team of experts, sleep is in fact incredibly important for your health and aids the process of healing
the damage that life brings you every day. In fact, it is just as
important (and perhaps even more important depending upon
where you find yourself physically and mentally) as eating right
and exercising well.

Statistically, we are sleeping less today than we did back
twenty-five to fifty years ago.[10] We pride ourselves on sleeping
less and brag about how little we can sleep and still function. But
the truth is, we aren't functioning, and without sleep we age pre-
maturely, our bodies break down and do not repair themselves,
our brains start to fog, our moods become unstable, and more.

Studies prove that a lack of sleep leads to weight gain. Did you
get that? According to the research, lack of sleep messes up your
appetite and hormones and causes you to be hungry when you
aren't.[11] Is it all in the brain? No. I said hormones. Sleeping can
help you with actual appetite regulation. So sleep and get skinny.

When we sleep, it impacts brain function. Lack of sleep

impairs cognition ("the mental action or process of acquiring knowledge and understanding through thought, experience, and the senses"[12]), limits our ability to concentrate, and impairs our productivity (the ability to get stuff done) and performance.[13] My doctors inform me that this includes bedroom function.

But here's the big one on sleeping: our amount and quality of sleep, experts believe, can actually have a major impact on our risks for flipping those genetic switches that lead to chronic diseases, including arthritis, diabetes, heart diseases, and mental illness.[14] This isn't just about your face sagging, your hair falling out, being tired and sluggish, or putting on the pounds.

How much sleep do you need? Some studies found that less than seven good hours (when you get your best rest, hit REM, and dream) leads to total physical and mental impairment.[15] In contrast, seven to eight hours of sleep per night leads to health and wellness.

WATER

Here's another revelation that seems obvious, but you likely are not anywhere close to following: you need to drink water. Hydration is important!

Water bottles are everywhere. Plastic ones on shelves are full of the clear stuff, and empty bottles in all shapes and sizes with all kinds of designs are designed to get you to buy. Water is not just a money-making monster, although it certainly is that. Hydration (meaning water, not Diet Coke or coffee) is essential to your health.

When I asked the people closest to me whether or not they drank water, the answers were sketchy. I got a lot of yes replies, of course. But when I asked, "How much?" the stops, stares, and shudders told the story. It seemed that everyone I knew, even the ones who looked healthy, took drinking water for granted. Water is crucial, and nearly all of us fail to consume enough to help the body do what it needs to do!

Here's what we know: around 65 percent of the average adult's body is made up of water.[16] That is a lot of water. It is in your organs and everywhere else. Your body is a big bottle of water. If there is so much water in you, why do you need so much of it?

Your cells need water to function properly. Your organs need water to function properly. Your joints are lubricated by it. Your spinal cord is jacked without it. It regulates your body's temperature. You cannot digest well without it. (That means if you are constipated, it is not just because you are not getting enough fiber.)[17]

And then there is kidney function. Our kidneys filter around one hundred and thirty quarts of fluid a day. About two of those quarts happen when we urinate. The rest is in the bloodstream.[18] Water is essential for the kidneys to work right. If the kidneys are not working right, waste and excess toxic fluid build up and jack us up. Our organs are damaged, and we get urinary tract infections, kidney stones, and more. Water has a tremendous and positive impact on all of this!

When you drink more water, your blood pressure will be positively impacted. Asthma is impacted. Skin problems are impacted.[19] By drinking more water, I noticed I am thinking clearer, I am having an easier time in the men's room, my headaches are gone, and my inflammation is improved. Try it.

THE FOUR PROCESSES

K. C. Craichy told me that every disease has up to four processes going on (or in the case of methylation, not going on) for the disease to advance, including oxidation, inflammation, glycation, and methylation.[20]

Oxidation refers to "the loss of an electron by an atom or molecule."[21] If an enzyme or an essential protein or any such critical molecule loses an electron, it can cause significant damage. Free radicals, atoms with one or more unpaired electrons that are produced by natural body processes or introduced by toxins or pollutants, are the cause of oxidation. Antioxidants, such as beta carotene and vitamin C, counteract and immobilize free radicals. If the body does not have sufficient antioxidants to deal with the free radicals, the free radicals damage healthy cells by altering their chemical structure. It has been noted that "many body processes can easily be disrupted in this way, leading to widespread damage and aging."[22]

Inflammation, as we have discussed, can be a good, healthy process by which the body heals itself. However, inflammation can also be a bad thing. Signs of inflammation include redness, heat, and pain. There is also a type of low-grade inflammation that can permeate the entire body; it does not result in typical inflammation symptoms and can only easily be detected by means of blood tests.[23] Research continues to demonstrate a positive link between inflammation and conditions such as cancer, diabetes, cardiovascular disease, and Alzheimer's disease.[24]

Glycation is the "bonding of a sugar molecule, such as glucose or fructose, to a protein or lipid molecule, without the controlling action of an enzyme."[25] Glycation produces molecules with damaged, distorted structures that produce large amounts of free radicals, those pesky atoms we already discussed when we learned about oxidation. The damaged molecules are known as advanced glycation end-products (AGEs).[26] AGEs "can clog the very small blood vessels...throughout the body, especially in the kidneys, eyes, heart, and brain.... Accumulation of AGEs can wreak cellular havoc, contributing in turn to oxidative stress, chronic inflammation, and premature aging. It is also associated with many chronic diseases and conditions, including insulin resistance, type 2 diabetes, cardiovascular disease, Alzheimer's, Parkinson's, rheumatoid arthritis, cataracts, cancer, and kidney disease."[27]

Methylation is "a fundamental detox process occurring constantly in every cell" that is necessary for cell function. Methylation, chemically speaking, "is the process of moving a methyl group—CH3—around in a cycle." For this to occur, the raw material for the required methyl groups and certain catalysts, such as B vitamins, need to be present. When they are not present, it "causes a blockage to the cycle leading to serious health issues." It has been noted that when the methylation process is working well, it helps the body fight carcinogenic toxins and repair damaged DNA; however, when the process is not working well, it results in degeneration.[28] Studies show that "changes in DNA methylation patterns have been observed in association with CVD [cardiovascular disease], inflammation, autoimmune diseases, infections and cancer."[29]

If we can deal with the four processes nutritionally, then theoretically the disease cannot progress. We can address the four processes nutritionally by incorporating foods with things such as omega-3 fatty acids, which control many basic cell functions and may help prevent and treat coronary artery disease, arthritis, cancer, and other inflammatory and autoimmune disorders, and vitamin D, which promotes the intestinal absorption of calcium and phosphorus. K. C. notes 85 percent of us are lacking in vitamin D and it is important to have your vitamin D levels checked during regular blood tests (ideal levels are thought to be 50 ng/dl to 75 ng/dl). The human body needs about 5,000 IU of D_3 a day, which is best taken with a fat food. K. C. Craichy said that if you eat a diet of sugar and fast foods, then you are going to feed the four processes. Over and over again, K. C. stressed to me simplicity and how easy I can make things for myself.[30]

If you are like me, you have been eating an undisciplined diet of convenience for many years. We usually go for what is easy to access and appeals to our taste buds, ignorant to the fact that what we eat significantly impacts our bodies and minds. The old saying of "You are what you eat" is not far from the truth. This particular axiom showed up in the writings of nutritionist Victor Lindlahr in the 1920s. He said it this way: "Ninety percent of the diseases known to man are caused by cheap foodstuffs. You are what you eat." [31]

Our diets are more about psychology than physiology. I understand how we have been misled by food developers, marketers, and retailers. It is time to take back control of our food, bodies, health, and longevity.

I am learning to take care of my body, the temple of God's Spirit. When God said that the Spirit lives within the believer, He could have said that our body (rather than a temple) was His Spirit's house. I think we might have kept it up better, considering how we would want His house to look! And I am not just talking about the outside.

Have you ever known someone whose house looked great on the outside, but when you went inside, you wondered who in the world would live there? When I was in high school, I agreed to watch the house of a couple from church. They were going on a two-day trip and needed someone to house-sit and mind their dogs. All I had to do to earn some extra cash was drop by, take the dogs out, and feed them and such. What could go wrong?

The couple wore nice clothes and drove brand-new Cadillacs, and their house was impressive on the outside. I figured their house would be a great place to throw a legendary house party, so I planned it all out. I needed the party to happen the first night because that would give me a day to clean and put things back into order. After my second job, I raced to the house. I had purchased all the food and drinks, loaded them into my car, and asked my buddies and their friends to meet me at the house. I was running late, and upon my arrival, I found my twelve friends sitting in the drive and waiting on me.

With bags of chips and drinks in hand, I struggled to the door. My hands were full, so I asked my girlfriend to grab the keys and open the door. As the door swung wide, my first thought was that I wouldn't let my dog live in this place!

The front hallway had at least five or six pairs of shoes lying around. The kitchen trash overflowed the bin and rested on the floor. The counters were covered with food boxes, open cans, and at least a week's worth of dishes with food stuck to them. The sink was full and nasty. The living room looked like a war zone. The beds were unmade, and dirty clothes were everywhere. I won't even talk about the toilet in the guest bathroom—think science experiment. Obviously, the party was a disaster.

People often treat their bodies the same way—great on the outside and a disaster within. Our bodies are supposed to be a shrine for the Spirit. I believe God intended for our temples to be a sacred place, where the Spirit lives, yes, but where we worship and honor Him by how we treat it.

When I started really learning about my body, discovering its power and how God made it and learning what it was to take care of it, I discovered that by respecting it I am honoring God in the process. That may sound a little super-spiritual, but consider all God put behind its design and then consider how much we take it for granted and abuse it. Many of us treat our cars better than we do our bodies. We protect our money better than we protect our bodies.

Realizing that my body is not my own, that God bought it with a price, and that He intends for His Spirit to take up residence within it helped serve as one of the greatest motivators to start looking at my body differently and to start taking care of it as I should.

Imagine if you were twenty pounds lighter. Imagine if your skin rebounded. Imagine if you were able to slow down the aging clock. By taking small, simple steps in the right direction, you can start looking, feeling, and doing as if you were twenty years younger! This isn't just hype or positive thinking. It is absolutely and totally possible, and I will tell you that if you do what I have done, you will see the same kind of results. And with the Spirit living inside you, you not only look and feel better, but you are infused with a power to do what you never thought possible! You will be stronger. You will be smarter. You will move easier. You will look good, live great, and love well. Let's do this!

Chapter 8

HEALING FROM THE INSIDE

S EVERAL YEARS AGO I boarded a plane and flew to Israel to produce a documentary on olive trees. The land of Israel has gone through so much industrialization over the last decades, and with so many of Israel's young people moving away, the country has gone through somewhat of an evolution. Technology, science, and other influences have, as many believe, moved the sacred things away from a central position of importance in the hearts and minds of some of the people. Development and industrialization has given rise to a reduction of land available for agriculture. In Israel, there is not much land to go around.

Some organizations in Israel are planting olive trees to preserve olive groves and marketing to a worldwide audience how people who love Israel can adopt an olive tree in the name of their family in one of the prominent groves. I hosted one such show. I had been to the country before. After my father died, a monument was presented to honor him for his life's work for the country, specifically for evangelical Christians. On that visit, I was taken into the hills of the American Independence Park, which extends from Beit Shemesh to Bar Giora on the southwestern side of the Judean Hills. This park honors the deep ties between America and Israel. I was there to dedicate a limestone monument inscribed by Pastor Benny Hinn and to plant my own olive tree.

I was back again, only this time on a ten-day excursion in the hot Israel sun producing a documentary. We captured footage all across the country—on the Mount of Olives, in Nazareth, all through the Holy City, at the Wailing Wall, on the Temple Mount, and even in the Garden of Gethsemane. Our days were full. I was up at 5:00 a.m. and in the makeup chair by 6:30. Production days were long and hard. It was around the fifth day that I became severely ill.

ROADSIDE VENDORS AND REGRET

On the way back to my hotel one night, I asked the driver to pull over to a roadside vendor selling local foodstuffs. It had been a long day. I had not eaten much, and I was starving. We pulled up to a roadside vendor, and I could smell the scent of something good drifting through the window. The driver stopped, turned around, and asked in broken English, "Are you sure?"

I said, "Yeah, I'm famished." I had traveled quite a bit by this time in my life. I had been to Africa, India, Brazil, and Central America. I had eaten at nearly every corner bodega in New York City. I know the rule of thumb about eating strange foods from roadside vendors. But I thought, "This is Israel! If there was ever

God's country, this is it!" In about three minutes I had something with lamb and onions in it.

I said a quick prayer. My friend and traveling companion, Pastor Otoniel Font, said, "God help you in about three hours from now."

I replied, "This is sanctified and covered by the blood!" (I don't think I added "of the Lamb" as a play on words, but I am pretty sure I thought it.)

Three hours later the pastor's prophecy came true. I found myself in cold sweats, and I crawled into a scalding hot tub in my hotel room just to stop the shivering. I remember lying there thinking, "I'm going to die, and they will say that a lamb killed me. God is teaching me a lesson for making light of the blood." I'm serious. The craziest things go through your mind when you think you're dying! When I tell you I was sicker than sick in a tub in Jerusalem, I'm telling you that I felt as if death would be better than the pain I was suffering in my body. I shivered. I shook. My digestive system was rebelling by every possible method. I was absolutely miserable.

My point of sharing this story is not the depiction of my plight in my hotel room but what happened to me afterward. The next day I slowly recovered. The production crew had thankfully let everyone off for the weekend, so I had Saturday and Sunday to recover. On Saturday I ate nothing, naturally. I felt like a truck had run over me. My insides were turned inside out! There was nothing inside me. I was only able to get down a little water. Saturday rolled by. I woke on Sunday, around 1:45 a.m., to the Muslim call in Israel. I looked over at the digital clock in my room. I realized I had slept all day and into the night.

As the Muslim cry painted the background, mesmerizing and hypnotic, I thought how amazing the devotion of these people was. I wondered who in America would be praying with such religious obedience. Suddenly, my attention shifted to something else. I had the most amazing surge of energy. I sat right up in the bed. I felt as though I had been energized by the prayer call. I knew that couldn't be it, so I thought, "Man, it is amazing what some really good sleep will do for you." I swung my feet over the bedside, started to step onto the floor, and paused, because instinctively I knew once my feet hit the floor I would feel the usual agony from my ongoing inflammation.

Only this time, it was different. My feet hit the marbled floor and I felt…good. I stood—no pain in my joints. I walked— no pain in my knees. I lifted my hands, made a fist, and then relaxed my hands again—no stiffness, no inflammation, no pain. I couldn't believe my senses. I opened a bottle of water, drank it fast, lay on the couch, and drifted off to sleep. When I woke, the only thing I could think about was the fact that in the middle of the night my inflammation and pain was gone. I thought maybe I had a dream that it was so because I was in pain again. My heart sank. But as I stood, there was no pain or inflammation in my hands, joints, or knees. But my neck was killing me. Then I remembered I had slept on the couch. I don't think I was ever happier to wake having slept wrong with the pain to prove it. But there was no inflammation!

I thought, "God has healed me! Here I am doing this olive tree thing, and God looked down and blessed me." I immediately vowed to plant a hundred olive trees of my own. A little dramatic, I know, but the craziest things go through my mind when the craziest things happen to me. I am sure you can relate.

Upon returning home and back to normal life, I was on cloud nine. I felt good for the most part. I didn't tell anyone I was healed, mainly because within twenty-four hours of arriving home, it seemed as though the inflammation was creeping back. And indeed, it was. Within a week the pain was back in full swing. It wasn't full-tilt, like I would experience later, after returning to the States from the Congo. But this event left an indelible mark in my brain that I would revisit upon the discovery of just how much is going on in our gut and how our gut leads to so much of what causes breakdown in our bodies over time.

IT ALL BEGINS WITH YOUR GUT

All disease begins in the gut.

—HIPPOCRATES[1]

It all begins with your gut. Your gut is the "biggest immune system organ," as noted by Donald Kirby, MD, the director of the Center for Human Nutrition at the Cleveland Clinic.[2]

They call it leaky gut syndrome. And yet, with an ever-increasing mountain of evidence and supportive data and doctors all over the world starting to chime in, this condition might very well be what causes chronic inflammation throughout the body.[3]

It is suggested that prolonged and chronic inflammation could lead to everything from chronic fatigue syndrome, rheumatoid arthritis, lupus, migraines, multiple sclerosis, and some believe, even autism in children.[4]

Even though much of the medical community is struggling to give solid credence or support to this discovery, the entire natural wellness and alternative medicine arena is standing on the rooftops and shouting about it.[5] The biggest issue is that it is hard to really diagnose. Because there is not a real solid way to test for it, mainstream acceptance remains elusive. But opinion is changing as more and more experts come forward with story after story of just how much the gut contributes to overall health.

As we discussed, our digestive system's barrier is like a window screen—the air flows through, but the screen keeps the flies out.

Nutrients the body needs are like air. They pass through the tiny holes by design. The holes keep out larger particles that are bad for you. With leaky gut syndrome, the window screen is a mess. The holes become larger, and all kinds of junk passes through along with the good nutrients—viruses, undigested food particles, and other things, all leaking into your bloodstream. When this happens, it triggers an immune response, which if sustained, perhaps leads to the diseases listed above.

I had all the symptoms of leaky gut syndrome. I discovered the factors that trigger the condition: bad diet; medication and antibiotics; stress and anxiety; sugar; overgrowth of yeast in the stomach; chemicals in what we eat, wear, and wash with; and gluten, a protein that many are finding they are actually allergic to, found in wheat, rye, and barley.

Suddenly, I understood: eating equals inflammation. It was like clockwork. Every time I ate, I would feel it within days. Sometimes it was there, and sometimes it was gone. I could almost predict it. Over time it seemed that I was growing weaker. My skin looked different. My hair was thinning fast. I had heartburn all the time. I felt bloated, my joints ached, and I had a low-grade fever. There were rashes that appeared and then went away.

After I wrapped the production in the Congo and returned to see a rheumatologist, who put me on high-powered, toxic medications, I started my journey to look deeper. But then something happened that set me on the path to determine how I could attack what was going on in my body and gave me some real traction.

I was in the office, and my HR director came in looking like death warmed over. He had this look of despair on his face, and he said, "Sir, I'm going home. I'm trying to fight it, but three people have already left throwing up. I can't hold out any longer." I told him to go because I could not afford to get sick. I make my living in front of the camera, producing television programming for some of the largest brands, and I realized that if I was out of commission, the company itself would nearly be out of commission. Well, it was too late. In the tight confines of our offices and production studios, someone brought in a bug, and we had a full-fledged flu epidemic in the halls of Legacy Worldwide. Within seventy-two hours, twenty-three of forty-five staff members were out sick. And then it hit me. It was not as bad as Israel, but it wasn't far from it.

Something amazing happened though. In the days following my "purge," the inflammation was gone again. If empty gut equals inflammation gone, then I must have leaky gut. It was so simple. So I began the journey to find out everything I could. I also thought that if I could cause my gut to become distressed, then there must be something that I could do to heal it.

My initial research did not produce much. The conventional route, talking to conventional doctors, produced nothing. My conversations with most alternative wellness folk were equally empty in terms of what I was looking for: practical steps.

In most cases, I was told the obvious: there is no cure for leaky gut because no one has been able to confirm it exists. Those who were inclined to give it serious consideration offered the basics, which, while helpful, were only good once you healed the gut. Nevertheless, it is worth mentioning for later on: Switch to an anti-inflammatory diet. Cut out dairy and gluten. Do away with sugar entirely (if possible). No alcohol. My new diet consisted of essential fatty acids found in fish and nuts, lots of vegetables (especially the leafy green stuff), high-fiber foods (but nothing with gluten), and my favorite, sauerkraut. (Fermented foods are really good for you. It's all about healthy bacteria in your gut.)

But to heal the gut? Where did I begin?

HEALING THE GUT

For most, the issue is with candida, a fungus and form of yeast that in overabundance wreaks havoc in the walls of your intestines.[6] It is a big contributor to leaky gut. To combat candida, we have to build up the friendly bacteria. Supplements can help, which I detail at ZoeLogics.com if you would like more specific findings.

To deal with the candida issue, immediately activate a no-sugar diet and all the good eating I detailed above and in the back of this book. Cut down to only one cup a day of the more complex carbohydrates, like potatoes. This will help prevent the candida from growing, and with this one-two punch, the candida will die.

Also, coconut oil is amazing. One spoon a day goes a long way. Organic coconut oil is said to poke holes in the yeast cell wall and will cause it to die, promoting wellness in your body.

In addition to introducing gut-healing foods into the system, you can also add a probiotic, glutamine, and glutathione. I provide several great examples of the exact products that I took, also at ZoeLogics.com.

But nothing worked to attack the issue of my gut health better than something that we've known about, the Bible has talked about, and people have practiced for over two thousand years: fasting. Yes, fasting.

Having discovered what happened to me when I got sick and, for lack of a better term, purged the toxins from my body, I learned to recover my health. I realized I had to remove the source of the degradation to my health. Once you identify your own triggers, it will become obvious that you need to remove them!

Every time my system was empty, it was as if my body reset itself. I figured if I could reset my body by cleansing my gut, I could initiate my body's God-given ability to heal itself.

Everywhere I researched, including God's Word, I found that there is no faster way to push down the inflammation in our body than fasting. Through the process of fasting, we restart our system. We in essence empty the bowl and allow our digestive system a period to rest from its work and time to heal. I discovered that fasting is and was used in modern and ancient cultures alike to jump-start the healing process within the body. And remarkably, hardly anyone in conventional medicine is even talking about it!

And watch this—fasting is how we trigger a reset to our soul/spirit battle.

The process for clinics and hospitals to break an addiction is to starve that addiction. The Bible talks about fasting, which is the same thing. It is what Daniel did. Jesus did it too. Pastors call congregations to this, and it was part of the early days of my journey. Some people of faith fast weekly and monthly for psychological or spiritual reasons or just for general health reasons. When Jesus fasted, it was because of the Spirit leading Him. I'm calling on you to fast, but there needs to be some way to starve the soul and launch the spirit. We need to starve the soul of whatever has caused it to rage out of control.

Jesus taught us of the power of prayer and fasting.

> Jesus said to him, "If you can believe, all things are possible to him who believes." Immediately the father of the child cried out and said with tears, "Lord, I believe; help my unbelief!" When Jesus saw that the people came running together, He rebuked the unclean spirit, saying to it: "Deaf and dumb spirit, I command you, come out of him and enter him no more!" Then the spirit cried out, convulsed him greatly, and came out of him. And he became as one dead, so that many said, "He is dead." But Jesus took him by the hand and lifted him up, and he arose. And when He

had come into the house, His disciples asked Him privately, "Why could we not cast it out?" So He said to them, "This kind can come out by nothing but prayer and fasting."
—MARK 9:23–29

By fasting, not only are we resetting our gut and preparing our body for repair, but we are simultaneously starving the cravings of our soul-led desires and allowing our spirit to rise within us. I could write an entire chapter just on fasting and its benefits in the soul/spirit battle within us, but for now we will stay focused on how fasting initiates healing in the gut and does a lot for the mind, as they are very much connected.

THE GUT–BRAIN CONNECTION

Dr. Leaf has written about the gut–brain connection. She notes that even though we must eat to survive, eating is also "a highly emotional and metacognitive event." Consider how food is often an integral part of social gatherings and celebrations. Dr. Leaf points out that "the joy of preparing a meal and sharing it with people is incredibly powerful, and incredibly therapeutic." Meals can be a source of either positive or negative emotions, and emotions affect the body's digestive system. She further states, "Our gastrointestinal tract (GI tract) is very sensitive to our emotions, since it is connected to the brain's hypothalamus, which controls both the feelings of satiety and hunger and deals with our emotional state of mind. The mind and the gut are acutely interconnected, and thus happiness, joy, and pleasure, as well as anger, anxiety, sadness, and bitterness, for example, trigger a physical reaction in your digestive system."[7]

Dr. Leaf also warns against eating when angry or to mask other negative feelings, as well as ignoring what our digestive system is telling us. In addition, she says, "Toxic thinking and emotions…can affect the movement and contractions of the GI tract, cause inflammation, make you more susceptible to infection, decrease nutrient absorption…give you indigestion and heartburn by increasing the acid in your stomach, make you feel nauseous, cause existing digestive issues such as stomach ulcers to worsen, and agitate your colon in a way that gives you diarrhea, constipation and/or extreme bloating," among other things.[8]

I began my fast with straight lemon water for twenty-four hours. I then sipped only bone broth for the next forty-eight hours. So for three straight days I hadn't introduced *any* food into my system. I also incorporated prayer, worship, managed stress, and very light exercise (walking and non-spiritual yoga) into my routine. I was feeling somewhat weak, but by day three my inflammation was completely gone!

On day four I added only green leafy vegetables into my diet, while remaining on the bone broth and lemon water. I threw myself into worship and prayer and voraciously immersed myself in the Word, while still managing my daily work and light exercise. On day five I was feeling like a million bucks. My gut was noticeably shrinking, though that had nothing to do with my gut healing. There is nothing like losing some weight along the way. So on day five I introduced fermented foods, such as homemade kefir yogurt (which you can learn how to make on my website) and began a regimen of glutamine supplements, vegetables, coconut oil, and of course, my favorite, lemon water. As always, I stayed in prayer and the Word, which I committed to making a staple of the rest of my days, along with management of stress and light exercise.

On day six I repeated day five but also introduced some organic coffee into my morning routine, but with no real dairy, meaning no cream, and no sugar. Instead, I used a teaspoon of organic coconut oil and two teaspoons of grass-fed butter. I whipped it all in a blender, and let me tell you—it was amazing. Try it.

On day seven I splurged a little. It was time to rest! I continued everything previously mentioned, but I had some grass-fed chicken.

While this regimen worked for me and got me started on my road to complete recovery, it is only one of many plans you might find helpful for you. The bottom line is that it is time for you to do *something*. As the old saying goes, "The definition of insanity is doing the same thing over and over again and expecting different results."

You have been sick long enough. It's time to do what I did and let the experience of being sick and in pain be the trigger to move you in the right direction. Let's move in the direction of God. He cures.

When we start to detox, by fasting or otherwise, we start to realize what a toxic world we really live in! It isn't interested in us finding our vision, our gift, and our purpose. It is geared toward taking our money. That's it. I believe it is driven by a force that wants to blind us, get us sick, and take us down.

GOING 1ONONE

Trying to discover how God cures inspired me to start the *1onONE* show a few years ago. I wanted to have guests who could provide in-depth research and knowledge of an issue, a need, or controversial truths. But it was my goal to find a solution to what leads to our struggle as children of God. And when it came to health issues, I have been privileged to get to know firsthand what the problems are in our food system and diets. But even more importantly, I have learned about how we can fix some of our own health brokenness. The experience of producing this program, which is still going strong, was one of my motivating factors in the concept for *God Cures*. I want to share with you some of what I discovered from some good friends of mine along the way.

I have had the privilege of getting to know and interview Dr. Joel Wallach, author of the international best seller *Dead Doctors Don't Lie*. He is a pioneer in human health and nutrition. As a biomedical research pioneer, Dr. Wallach spent more than forty years observing and researching the effects of individual nutrients on health. Dr. Wallach says he was able to pinpoint the cause of many diseases as nutrient deficiencies through extensive research. Disease can be cured, ailments eliminated, and life prolonged simply by giving the body what it needs to heal itself! Today he is renowned for his groundbreaking research on the health benefits of selenium and other minerals. He is revolutionizing the way we look at health care.[9]

Like many of the experts I have invited to share with us during this journey, Dr. Wallach first became interested in health and nutrition and solutions to health challenges because of a real health crisis he was experiencing. Dr. Wallach told me that when he was four years old, he began developing symptoms of what today we would call Tourette syndrome. He was having tics in his facial nerves. Dr. Wallach says the symptoms continued until he was nine years old, and medical doctors couldn't identify the problem or offer any solution.[10]

Every morning, Dr. Wallach had chores to complete at the family farm before going to school, including feeding alfalfa tablets fortified with vitamins and minerals to the calves. He read the label and saw the list of vitamins and minerals. The next day at school he found a book called *The Nurse's Handbook*. He flipped through the index and found a listing for cramps. The book reported that cramps were caused by a calcium deficiency.

And the light went off—he knew there was calcium in the alfalfa pellets fed to the calves! The next morning, he threw the Cheerios from his cereal bowl to the chickens, poured those alfalfa tablets into his bowl with the milk, and started a routine. Dr. Wallach says that three days later his symptoms were gone! [11]

Obviously, Dr. Wallach has been on a quest to figure out how our bodies work since he was very young. Most nine-year-old kids aren't going to the library to find medical reference books!

I asked him why so many people are sick and unhealthy. He said that it is actually quite simple. He explained that we are sick because we are not giving our genes, DNA, RNA, and all of the end caps on our chromosomes the nutrition they need so that they can function the way the good Lord intended. He affirmed that we are made in God's image, but think about it— God doesn't experience the health problems we do. God doesn't have hemorrhoids, diabetes, or high blood pressure. [12]

Dr. Wallach explained that every vertebrate needs ninety essential vitamins, minerals, amino acids, and fatty acids. The Garden of Eden was the most fertile place on earth, and thus Adam and Eve could have all of their nutritional needs met. But we don't live in that world or that garden anymore. He articulated several examples of how our soil, rivers, and fertilization components have changed, and we are rarely, if ever, receiving the nutrients we need from the fruits and vegetables that we eat. We aren't made to have diabetes, heart disease, low thyroid function, and Alzheimer's disease, but we *are* routinely suffering from these diseases because our diets don't have the nutrients in them we need. [13]

Several things struck me during my discussions with Dr. Wallach. So many people have given in to whatever they are facing. A doctor has given them a prognosis, and it is not a good one. People have become defeated because of how they feel every day. I asked Dr. Wallach at the time of my first interview with him, "What can people do?"

Dr. Wallach began to articulate the cures for different diseases with proper vitamins and minerals to overcome the deficiencies causing the diseases. If ever there was corroboration of the precept that knowing and doing the truth can set us free, then what Dr. Wallach has discovered is proof positive that truth can change our lives forever! He said that we are misinformed when told that all we have to do is eat a well-balanced meal. Chiefly that is true because plants, fruit, and grains do not make many of the nutrients we need. Minerals have to come from the soil, and if that soil is depleted or overwrought with chemical fertilizers, then we won't receive all we need from the plants we eat. Dr. Wallach also has accumulated years of historical and cultural research to show why our soils are depleted.[14]

Dr. Joseph Christiano (Dr. Joe) has joined me in the *IonONE* studio many times over the years, and viewers of my program have clamored for more. Dr. Joe lives by the philosophy "Faithful caretaking of your body is an obligation, not an option."[15] I want to share some of his professional insights on how to heal our bodies from the inside out through the blood type diet. His book *Bloodtypes, Bodytypes and You* is an incredible guide to getting your eating habits on the path to transforming your body and health.

BLOOD TYPES AND FOOD

One of the foundational truths that Dr. Joe points out in his book is that our individual genetic makeup makes us different than just about anyone else. That may not be news to you, but what Dr. Joe puts forth is that because of our unique makeup, we each need to eat different foods! Obviously, as you can see from the title of his book, blood types are an easy indication or marker of those differences. We have types A, B, AB, and O.

When I interviewed Dr. Joe, he laid out a simple scenario. If four people with four different blood types all eat the same meal, about an hour after the meal they would all feel differently. One feels energized, one feels a bit lethargic, one has a bit of discomfort in their colon, and the fourth is somewhere in between. Think about the last time you shared a large meal with your friends. Did everyone react to the meal the same way? What Dr. Joe did was to take a closer look for us.[16]

He says that an hour or so after we eat we should be feeling well, and if we are not, then our body is trying to tell us something. And we should be listening. Dr. Joe says that God designed us at the blood and cellular levels to run best while ingesting foods that have compatible antigens. So it is not just about eating healthy; it is about eating "correctly."[17]

Dr. Joe researched fifty-two hundred individuals with different blood types, ages, genders, and diseases. What he found was that many of them had developed a disease at a premature age, and most could trace it to their blood type and what they had been eating. Thus, he confirmed that they could reverse some of the effects of their disease through changing their diets so the types of food they were eating were compatible with their blood type.[18]

Dr. Joe takes that axiom we mentioned earlier, "You are what you eat," and adds to it, "But it is also vitally important for you to eat what you are!" Each of us should eat a diet that is compatible with our blood type. We can begin to get an understanding of this important concept by taking a look at the animal kingdom. It is instinct that drives animals to eat. Lions are meat eaters. They won't be happy if you try to feed them a diet rich in fruits and vegetables. Other animals are vegetarian by instinct, and they will not eat meat. This is no accident. Instinct is a protective mechanism for all animals, including humans. Each blood type has different characteristics that allow it to eat, digest, and assimilate the food best for that group. Those with type O are blessed with strong stomach acid and powerful enzymes that can metabolize almost anything—even food not recommended for them. Types A, B, and AB must be more careful in their eating habits or suffer the consequences.[19]

What are these consequences? When you don't eat food compatible with your blood type, agglutination happens. Your body has antibodies that protect it from foreign invaders. Your immune system produces all kinds of antibodies to protect you and keep you safe from foreign substances. Each antibody is designed to attach itself to a foreign substance or antigen. When your body recognizes an intruder, it produces more antibodies to attack the invader. The antibody then attaches itself to the intruder, and a "gluing" effect (agglutination) takes place. In this way, the body can better dispose of these foreign invaders.[20]

> When it comes to eating foods that are not compatible with your blood type, this "gluing" effect can take place in the digestive system, joints, liver, brain or blood. Continual ingestion of foods not compatible to your blood type can cause havoc in your body systems. This agglutination of cells, or clumping, will eventually break down the function of that particular system and lead to health problems.[21]

You can see why I am interested in Dr. Joe's coaching and input. When you consider the many health problems that can occur, it is vitally important for us to pay attention to this kind of research! He also shares my interest in improving our lives holistically, body, soul, and spirit. My blood is type O, and Dr. Joe has told me I am predisposed to arthritis, which means that my diet can either fuel the arthritis or fight against it. If I am eating incompatible foods, then I am fueling disease, and if I am eating blood type–compatible foods, then I am fighting against disease and illness.

One thing Dr. Joe told me when we were discussing common symptoms of developing diseases has stuck with me: "We become accustomed to being toxic. I've seen it over and over." [22]

REAL CHANGE

I cannot stress enough the importance of the benefits that fasting has on the spirit and the soul. I believe it wasn't until incorporating fasting into my battle strategy that I began to see real change in the results. And let's face it, change is hard.

One of the people who has been a giant help and encouragement to me over the past ten years is Creflo Dollar. He was a gift from God at just the right time when I was facing crisis or sadness or victory. He has such wisdom and sensitivity to God's Spirit. He is constantly pointing people to Jesus and to God's Word for answers. But he has also taken the gifts he was given and sharpened and honed them to serve people. One of his attributes that I admire is how he helps people to change. He is great at helping people move from a commitment to change to actually taking the necessary steps to change and grow.

It is only appropriate that I include some of his words to help us in this journey. He wrote a book a few years back that has helped thousands of people: *8 Steps to Create the Life You Want: The Anatomy of a Successful Life*. One excerpt is spot on for our journey and the goal to live a life of wholeness of body, soul, and spirit:

> Have you ever desired to change, but felt you couldn't? Do you believe certain behaviors are impossible to change? The truth is, nothing is impossible with Christ. You have

at your disposal God's manual for life—His Word. It is the tool that will enable you to become completely whole and to accomplish your life's purpose.

Renewing your mind through meditation will lead you to success. Joshua 1:8 says that meditating on God's Word is the path to obtaining a prosperous life.... Meditation is not just going quietly "within" to find a state of tranquility and peace. It's using the Word of God as a tool to find peace and solutions in your life. To *meditate* means to ponder, think about, and turn something over in your mind until you get understanding. It is not emptying your mind of all thoughts. On the contrary, when you meditate on the Word of God, you focus your thoughts on Scriptures and allow God to speak to you and give you revelation knowledge....

Through meditation, you gain wisdom and knowledge from God's Word that you would otherwise not have access to. The message behind each Scripture is illuminated and begins to penetrate your heart, giving you knowledge you would have never gained on your own.

New thought patterns don't form overnight. Renewing the mind requires consistency and a plan of action. *Practicing* meditation will give you strength and knowledge to overcome negative thought patterns and live victoriously.... Romans 12:2 states we are transformed by the renewing of our minds. The Word of God is the mind renewal system God wants you to use in order to reprogram your thought process and access healthy emotions.[23]

Recovery can be a difficult process, and restoration can be a difficult process, but there are many aspects of recovery that can be simpler than we make them. As my different advisors share based on their research and experience, it is important to keep solutions as simple as possible. I detailed a sample plan in the appendix that should help you. You don't have to do exactly what

I did. In fact, I tried several different variations until I found the one that worked for me. Remember, you don't fail until you quit. If you find that one plan doesn't work for you, then simply back up and try a different road. Make a tweak to the plan, and customize it for what you're able to stick with—and then stick with it. The important thing on this journey is to get moving and stay in motion. You don't stop until you stop. Get it?

Chapter 9

DREAMING REAL DREAMS

MY MOTHER ONCE said she felt it was too late for her to do the things she really wanted to do. Many of us feel that way. Time moves on; opportunities seem lost. My mother had this sense that she had passed her prime. My mother, like me, struggled for many years following her divorce from my dad. Life sometimes has a way of beating every ounce of hope for the future out of us.

My mom is a fighter. She is one of the toughest people I've ever met. She is wildly creative, can sing like a canary, and is one of the most optimistic people you'll ever meet. When she was growing up, her father worked all the time. Her mother was a counselor, and when she wasn't working, she was cooking, cleaning, sewing, and doing everything else necessary to keep the church and home going. My mother, one of five kids, grew up fast. Her youngest baby brother passed away at twelve. She was married at eighteen and had two kids quickly. My father moved her to Okinawa during the Vietnam War. Then her world fell apart after the blizzard of 1978, which dropped nine feet of snow in South Bend, Indiana. It seemed perfectly fitting for such a dark, cold, desperate time in our lives as Mom and I loaded up a small U-Haul and drove to her parents' home seeking refuge after her marriage and our home fell apart.

My mom met a man not long after whom everyone thought was the knight in shining armor, but he quickly turned out to be an abusive drunk. One night after a week of immense abuse, my mother put me on a plane to go live with my father. Two weeks later, the man who had been living with us tried to kill my mother by running their car off a cliff. If the small sports car they were driving had not hit a tree root extended from the cliffside, my mother would have met Jesus too early. Within days, with the help of a great attorney and close friends, my mother was settled in an apartment of her own and away from Satan's grasp. Life since then has been full of rough spots for her. Nevertheless, she went on to marry again and gave me an amazing brother, Cameron, and sister, Briana, who mean the world to me.

NEVER TOO LATE

Time seems to just slip away. It moves so quickly. You set out with great plans and big dreams, and then one day you wake up, look back at the chaos in your wake, and think, "There's got to be more." My mom kept fighting and never stopped dreaming. But dreaming for many becomes that—just dreaming. For some reason, when life kicks your teeth in and time passes and opportunity is lost, you can stop believing that your dreams are even possible. We start thinking that we're too old, it's too late, and all that negative stuff that separates the would-be Mick Jagger at forty-five from the Mick Jagger who is still rockin' at seventy-four. Someone said, "But hey, he started early." Julia Child didn't publish her first big, successful book until she was almost fifty, and that made her a household name! Vera Wang didn't get started as a designer until she was forty. Stan Lee, the Marvel Comics icon, didn't start his empire until he was almost forty. Samuel L. Jackson, who needs no introduction, was forty-six when got his breakout role. Henry Ford revolutionized the world with the Model T car at age forty-five!

It is never too late to dream real dreams. And my mom's flame was still lit.

We were in the auditorium of Living Word Christian Center outside of Chicago, Illinois, where Bill Winston was sharing the Word with a packed-out house and teaching on his new book, *Faith and the Marketplace*, which reveals that as believers we fall in two categories or corporate offices: kings or priests. He shared that God wants us to effect transformation in our cities and in the nations, and that through His power operating through us, miracles will happen in the marketplace. This teaching catapulted my mother's thinking to the next level. Everything changed for my mother.

Bill Winston exposed my mother and me to a new reality, one she never heard in church growing up. When Jesus came, He demonstrated a new reality, not just teaching the disciples about heaven or hell but teaching that the kingdom of God is available to us as believers right here on earth. As we sat listening intently and taking copious notes, Bill Winston shared that my mom was a citizen of this kingdom—a kingdom without sadness, poverty, and fear and where abundance was available and lack was nonexistent.

My mom was reminded that inside her exists a power greater

than life's struggles, that the years lost are redeemed in Jesus. One day we will receive our heavenly reward. Jesus came down so that we could discover how to live heaven on earth, that our eyes might be open to see who we really are and who God sees us to be—His children, who are capable of doing exactly what He created us to do. Time wasn't lost. Opportunity wasn't wasted. God has a perfect plan for our life. Bill Winston showed us that God was calling for the restoration of an unbeatable team of kings and priests to bring faith back into the marketplace and to help believers discover God's design for kingdom living right here on earth.

My mom heaved a big sigh, looked at me with that look of excitement she gets when God is birthing a big idea inside of her, and said, "It ain't over until it's over. Let's go. I got things to get busy doing for the kingdom. If there's a King, I'm the queen in charge!" My mom heard the right word at the right time, and in less than an hour everything changed for her.

And it is never too late for you. Remember that Jesus spent thirty years getting ready, and the most impact He had was in His last three years on earth. My mother is now over sixty and getting ready to fly to Mumbai, India, to build an orphanage, a school, and hopefully a medical clinic. She has been on this journey with me, and she has realized that her battle with relationships, her struggle with depressive thoughts along the way due to letdowns and setbacks, and her strenuous fight with asthma were nothing but a distraction to close the temple to the Spirit of God and keep her from realizing that God put her here to impact the world for Jesus.

TIME TO THRIVE

As for me, I'm going to sing. I'm going to stand on a stage, and I don't care how many people are in the audience. I'll have a drummer, a lead guitar, and a rhythm guitar behind me. The devil can try to stop me, but I'm not going to stop until the voice God has given me belts out, "It's never too late."

> For what is your life? It is even a vapor that appears for a little time and then vanishes away.
>
> —JAMES 4:14

I want to thrive! I believe we can thrive. I think we are supposed to maximize the time that we have. I think that every single one of us is born with something amazing on the inside. We see this in Jeremiah, where the Lord said, "Before I formed you in the womb I knew you; before you were born I sanctified you" (Jer. 1:5). Everything God does, He does for a purpose. And that includes making us.

I'll never forget the first time I got up to sing. I was nine years old. I used to watch my mom sing, and I was like, I can do that! There was this fire in me to do it—just like my mom. I used to listen to her practice with these cassette tapes. She'd hit the notes, and then when she went off to work I'd pop in the cassettes and see if I could hit the notes too. I could! So I was ready. Strike up the band, Joe! Give me the mic!

I convinced my grandfather and my mom to let me get up in front of the church and give it a whirl. There was opportunity each Sunday for some spontaneous singer to stand and say, "Y'all pray for me while I try to sing this song." But I wasn't going to go out that way. I had seen Elvis in Vegas on TV just a few years before, and I was planning on strutting out and doing it his way. But when the moment came, the gift inside was overshadowed by a little boy who was a little too shy, and I ended up singing "Jesus Loves Me" from behind a plant, center stage.

Search for the word *destiny* on the Internet and you know what you'll find? Lots of sites talking about a game called *Destiny*. Then eventually you will stumble onto a site or two about karma, but at some point you'll want to come to a conclusion about what destiny means for you and your life. For me, it is the purpose, mission, the *vocation* God gifted me to accomplish in my time on earth. Of course, our final destiny is to be with God in heaven and to see Jesus face-to-face and no longer through a foggy window.

Music has always been a powerful presence in my life. It has been said, "Medicine heals the body, but music heals the soul." And it was Plato who said, "Music and rhythm find their way into the secret places of our soul."[1] How true!

In terms of worshipping God, there is much that has been said and written through the centuries. King David brought music front and center into the worship experience. Many saints through the years have written music specifically for the worship of God. Bach used to write a new choral anthem every week for his church! Martin Luther once made the comparison, "Next to the Word of God, the noble art of music is the great treasure in the world."[2]

Finding the thing you are good at—your destiny—can happen when you least expect it.

We are so busy that we can't see what is right in front of us. Not only did I love to sing as a child, but I was also very active in theater productions in school. I joined the theater productions but really shied away from public singing until my sophomore year, when I tried out for a role in *Bye Bye Birdie*. I won the lead male role. Unfortunately, my dad wouldn't let me take the part because I had a B in one of my classes. It emotionally scarred me for many years. I had been forced to walk away from something I really enjoyed. I abandoned signing.

Many years later I was thirty-seven and on a production shoot in Jacksonville, Florida, with a buddy, Mike Anderson. We were at a karaoke restaurant with three hundred people in the room. Mike was there to sing, and I was there to support him. But Mike secretly put me on the list. On my way to the bathroom, I heard my name over the PA system. "Must be a mistake," I thought. It wasn't. To everyone's surprise, I came out and hit every note, right on key, in "Lights" by Journey. Mike and his friends at the table were freaking out. Their expressions went from guarded laughter for the joke to utter shock. And the crowd of people just froze. I walked off the stage, and something felt different. I felt like I was right where I was supposed to be. I was home.

Fast-forward to a trip to Thailand. We were eating in a restaurant filled with about six hundred mostly European patrons, and there was a band playing. Then I heard my name called. Mike had done it again. He paid the band to ask me to come up and join them in a song! I went up, stepped to the microphone, and sang U2's "With or Without You." I remember the response. I was utterly mobbed when I stepped off the stage. I was stopped and congratulated countless times. Mike witnessed it too. We were both amazed. I had never truly accepted that my voice was any good. The feeling while I was singing that song was unique and powerful. Nothing had ever felt that good. It reminded me of when I gave my life to God and felt this absolute peace. Or when my first baby daughter was born. Those moments are pinnacles.

Sometimes what we are supposed to do in life is hiding right under our noses, and we don't see it because we are too busy. The devil places roadblocks in our way and robs us of our destiny.

Part of the attack that I was facing in my health was the enemy's strategy to shut down my voice for good. Less than a month after I sang in Thailand, I received my diagnosis of rheu-matoid arthritis.

GETTING THE BAND TOGETHER

I've been trying to build a band for four years. You know what the problem is when you're trying to build a band? Finding time to rehearse can be difficult, sure, but you can't rehearse until you have band members. So the *real* problem is finding the members of the band. For four years I've been running ads and calling people who work with musicians, and I even went to Nashville for two weeks. I hired a music producer to help me put together a band. It hasn't happened yet.

Part of the premise of this book and this journey I'm on is that, as I'm finally becoming happy, healthy, and whole, I'm also getting in touch with my dreams and gifts. That's what I pray and hope for you too. I pray you find your own song and your own band.

I believe everyone has a gift. A gift is different than a talent. Of course, there's all kinds of advice floating around: "Do what you love." "Find your passion, and it'll never seem like work." "Don't make your hobby your job." You are familiar with all those say-ings and catchphrases. But it's funny how all the experts, gurus, educators, counselors, entrepreneurs, business leaders, moms and dads, and pastors point to the idea that you have been pro-grammed by intelligent design and each of us has a specific role and gift. At the same time, many believe there's a master strategy against you. It has been cooked up in some supernatural realm. There's a place that you cannot see with your naked eye designed to keep you from unleashing your gift on this world.

So while I have had this desire to sing and do music since I was five years old, I feel as though throughout my life there have been forces working against me to ensure I could never share my music with the world. Yet I was born to sing. I was born to rock 'n roll.

Putting the band together hasn't been an easy thing for me. But there is a time and a place for everything, and you'll see for yourself that during this journey, God may do some providentially supernatural things to bring your dream and gift to fruition.

My friend and concert pianist Dino Kartsonakis once said, "God gave me the talent, and I endeavor to give it back to Him with each new idea."[3] This is true of any gift that the Creator puts in our lives. Using the gift God specifically designated for us sets up a special relationship with Him. We want to honor and glorify God through the use of our gifts.

Author Madeleine L'Engle wrote in her book *Walking on Water: Reflections on Faith and Art*, "To paint a picture or to write a story or to compose a song is an incarnational activity. The artist is a servant who is willing to be a birth-giver. In a very real sense the artist (male or female) should be like Mary, who, when the angel told her that she was to bear the Messiah, was obedient to the command. . . . I believe that each work of art, whether it is a work of great genius or something very small, comes to the artist and says, 'Here I am. Enflesh me. Give birth to me.'"[4]

It's *your* destiny.

This book, and its suggestions for a healthier lifestyle, is not intended to replace a physician's care for people who have been diagnosed with a medical issue. However, there are specific ideas that all those who consulted with me during this journey have taught me, and if those ideas are applied properly, they could change your life forever.

Remember how important it is to remove sugar from our diets, detox before changing our eating plan, get enough sleep, remove the bad stress as much as we can, drink more water, pay attention to our bodies, and know that we, ourselves, may be the best doctor. We live inside our own bodies, and no one else does. We need to care constantly for the body, soul, and spirit.

In finding your destiny, you feed the soul and the spirit. When the soul and spirit are healthy, the body follows. Feeding the body properly helps keep that part of your triune being in homeostasis, and together all things work for your maximum health.

Chapter 10

THE JOURNEY

I F WE LIVE long enough, most of us are likely to see our fair share of calamity, struggle, and strain that necessitates the believer's cry for the supernatural touch of God. This topic, the need for a miracle, was especially pressing for me. And I lobbied with great faith that the Master of the universe, the Potter who shaped the clay, the Alpha and the Omega, Abba Father would reach down and spring forth a miracle in me.

For reasons only He can explain, my journey to total healing, to discovering how He cures, would be one to walk out, detail, and provide as a road map for others like you.

Like Job on the ash heap, Satan would have had it that I cursed God and died. Nothing could have been further from the truth. Simultaneously, God in His infinite wisdom, mercy, and loving grace has allowed my experience to help many be led out of the darkness of sickness and disease and into the light where they can share their own stories of triumph over tragedy.

Many who traveled this journey with me, the journey to walk out God's cure for my life, experienced supernatural breakthrough of their own. In fact, some days I found myself wondering how others had reached breakthrough so fast, yet there I was still in the desert, crossing ever so slowly and painfully.

Regardless, I have learned that God doesn't change. The pathway to the outcome might be different and our time frames unalike, but this much is always the same: God cures.

GOD'S GOODNESS INCLUDES HEALING

This book has lifted the lid on the enemy's schemes; however, it also has practical steps to get well. But it is critical that you understand that regardless of all the practical steps and how long it took for me to get to the other side, it is God who cures, and He can do it in a supernatural way in your life today.

I was raised in the Pentecostal church. I was raised around Spirit-filled, tongue-talking, laying-on-of-hands people who believed and operated in the power and authority of God. I have seen people run the aisles, people fall out in the Spirit, and demons cast out, and I have felt a power consume my body, a feeling I cannot explain except to recite a passage from the second chapter of Acts.

I was raised to believe that God can do what is impossible in the eyes of man. He is able to do in the supernatural what man could not possibly achieve in the natural. I have seen the miraculous and witnessed countless testimonies of the phenomenon of God's power, and again, most of it I cannot explain away with logic.

But God's logic confounds the logic of man. How can the finite begin to understand the infinite?

> "For My thoughts are not your thoughts, nor are your ways My ways," says the LORD. "For as the heavens are higher than the earth, so are My ways higher than your ways, and My thoughts than your thoughts."
>
> —ISAIAH 55:8–9

I have sat at the feet of the late, great Lester Sumrall, seen the power of the laying on of hands by Leroy Jenkins, walked through the passages of healing in the Word with Daniel Kolenda, and witnessed the power of God flatten an entire auditorium with thousands slain in the Spirit as I stood just stage right of Pastor Benny Hinn. I know without question that God's power is *real.*

You woke up this morning, and you had the fight of your life. Whether in your body, your finances, your relationships, or some combination of the three, Satan is coming at you with everything he has, and it is stealing your sleep, robbing you of your happiness, and making you question the promises of God as you are holding out hope for a miracle.

Well, I believe that supernatural healing is real. And in this chapter, the word *healing* is not just referring to the process by which the body is restored at the cellular level; it is referring to the God kind of healing, meaning "complete restoration and wholeness."

We must understand that God desires to be our Father. A good father provides and takes care of his children with all the resources he has at his disposal. So it is with God, our heavenly Father! Everything that He has is made available to His children because He is good and wants the best for His children. This provision of goodness from God includes healing of all kinds: spiritual, mental, and physical.

Jesus Christ was sent to redeem humanity and bring us back into the family of heaven so that God can be our Father and we can be His children. Jesus said in John 14:6, "I am the way, the truth, and the life. No one comes to the Father except through me." The word *comes* means "to make one's appearance before someone."[1] We cannot make our appearance before God as our Father without Jesus Christ preparing the way, revealing the truth that we can be God's children, and giving us divine access to eternal life with Him.

With this truth of Jesus Christ providing us access to God as our Father in mind, I would like to give you three ways to access the provision of healing He has made available to you as His child.

1. Know that God loves you enough to heal you.

It says in 1 John 4:19, "We love Him, because He [God the Father] first loved us." If you can settle in your mind that God already loves you, it takes the stress and pressure away of trying to perform to earn healing from Him. Through His eternal love for you, He has already provided healing of all kinds to you through His Son, Jesus. You do not have to earn a gift that has already been given.

2. Believe that God loves you enough to heal you.

You and I can do nothing to earn God's love and His provision of healing for us. God, being the loving Father that He is, would never express His love toward His children by giving them a sickness or disease. God does not have sickness or disease to give anyone because He does not have it to give. The Word of God says in James 1:17, "Every good gift and every perfect gift is from above, and comes down from the Father of lights, with whom there is no variation or shadow of turning." God only gives good and perfect gifts to His children. You must believe and be fully convinced that good and perfect gifts come from our Father, who will never change His mind about giving His children the best that He has!

3. Receive that God loves you enough to heal you.

In order to receive the gift of God's love, you and I have to take full possession of it. As a human being, you are made up of three parts: spirit, soul, and body. The real you is not your body, but it is your spirit, which possesses a soul. Your body is simply the house that you live in as you exist on planet Earth. The real you is made in the image and likeness of God, who is Spirit (Gen. 1:26–27; John 4:24). Since you were made to be just like God, He created you first and foremost as a spirit being, and you possess a soul (mind, will, and emotions) and have expression in this physical world through the body.

Healing is a part of the gift you received through Jesus Christ. You received Jesus into your spirit the day you accepted Him as your Lord and Savior. In John 10:10, Jesus says, "The thief does not come except to steal, and to kill, and to destroy. I have come that they may have life, and that they may have it more abundantly." The word *life* means "the absolute fullness of life that belongs to God."[2] It means "God's life." This God-life that Jesus has given you is put into your spirit. Now you must activate your soul (mind, will, and emotions) by renewing it with the promises from God's Word on healing (Rom. 12:1–2). You have to purposely think on God's promises on healing and keep your thoughts in line with those promises. As you do, your body will begin to change and manifest the healing that is on the inside of your spirit. Through this process of thinking on God's promises of healing that are already in your spirit, your soul is activated to agree with who you are in Jesus Christ, and your body will change and display the real you—healed, whole, and delivered. I believe in a supernatural God with supernatural power who wants to do something supernatural in your life right now.

GOD HEALS, AND GOD CURES

When you give it all up to the Master, when you call upon His name, when you rest in His mighty arms, when you surrender it all to Him, something truly miraculous can and *will* happen. I want you to agree with me that healing is possible. In fact, in just a moment, we are going to pray together for just that—God's cure for you right now. God heals, and God cures. His power to deliver you is available right now.

When I began this journey, Satan had me believing that sickness is what I deserved. Guilt and shame from my past had opened the doorway for the enemy to gain a stronghold in my mind—the place where nearly all battles in this life are fought and won.

I want you to follow me as I lean on the declarations of God's supernatural power and healing and His cure for us all:

> *Father, I thank You for Your love, I thank You for Your grace, and I thank You for Your power. As I humble myself before You, Lord, I ask that You forgive me and cleanse me as I surrender all to You. I surrender my will, my wants, my hopes, my dreams completely to You, Lord.*
>
> *Father, I thank You for the gift You planted in me, and I recognize right now that You created me for a purpose and that You marked my steps for destiny, that the world will see the ever-increasing eternal love that You have in Your heart for Your children.*

I thank You for what Jesus did at the cross, that His blood was shed for my sin. Lord, I receive the salvation made available to me, and I confess with my mouth that Jesus Christ is Lord over my life.

I declare that I am not defeated. I exercise the authority You have given me, and with my mouth I decree what it says in 1 John 4:4—greater is He who is in me than he who is in the world!

Father, the same Spirit who raised Jesus from the dead lives in me, and I know that, as Your Word says, Your favor surrounds me today as a shield.

My mouth is open, Lord, and I speak wisdom, filled with understanding, and I ask for an abundant supply from You today, God, just as it says in James 1:5.

I stand in agreement with Your Word, God, for my divine health and my divine healing. I am not sick, I am not broke, my relationships are whole, my mind is clear—and Lord, today my steps are ordered by You!

I thank You for supernatural strength today! I thank You for supernatural encouragement! I thank You for supernatural increase!

I rebuke any attack in my body, any attack in my finances, any attack against my family, and any attack that would attempt to set itself up against Your promises for my life, which are yes and amen!

Let every mountain in my way be moved. Let the troubled waters in my life be still. Let Your peace envelop me. Lord, let Your joy that is unmovable and full of glory fill my heart.

Lead me, Lord. Allow Your Holy Spirit to fill me and lead me as I follow You and Your will for my life.

I expect that today will be the first day of the best days of my life. My past is in my past, my future is before me, and I will walk in the supernatural power and dominion that You have given to me as a son (or daughter) of the Most High King! In Jesus's name I declare this. Amen.

I want to thank you for taking this time with me, investing yourself in my story, and allowing me to share my life, my experience, my understanding, and my wisdom and impart to you knowledge that will help you write your own experience.

This journey has been a tough one. God has sustained me. My pain and desire to get well, get back to normal, discover a new normal, and help profile how to escape the clutches of Satan have all served as motivators to make it through. But what drove me most—and what has kept me fighting—were the words my son said to me and his mother that one fateful day, the day he told us that he questioned the existence of God. But here is what we know:

> Draw near to God and He will draw near to you.
> —JAMES 4:8

> And when I am lifted up from the earth, I will draw everyone to myself.
> —JOHN 12:32, NLT

Regardless of where things are with you, your body, your finances, and your family, it all belongs to God. He knows what's going on. God is keeping track, and He is watching over His word to perform it: "I am watching to see that my word is fulfilled" (Jer. 1:12, NIV).

When I gave God what I was carrying, when I surrendered my health struggle, my shame of bad parenting, the guilt of my past, my unforgiveness, my fear of loss, and something I love and cherish so much—my son—all to Him, that is when God's power became the most evident. It was almost as if at my lowest, God became my Highest.

> And He said to me, "My grace is sufficient for you, for My strength is made perfect in weakness." Therefore most gladly I will rather boast in my infirmities, that the power of Christ may rest upon me.
>
> —2 Corinthians 12:9

Hope

A few weeks ago we sat as a family around the dinner table. It had been a while since we were all together. All my children were home: Makaela, my oldest girl; my son Avery; my other daughters, Sydney and Lexi; and my son Mason. I was tired, hungry, and ready to dive right in. Nathalie had prepared lasagna, and it was piping hot. I wasn't going to wait. I grabbed a spoon, dove into the pan, navigated a healthy portion onto my plate, and grabbed my fork for the first bite. What happened next was remarkable. Before my fork made its way to my mouth, my son Mason, the one who had shared with me and my wife that he was "searching" and curious about the possibility of God's existence, put his hand on my shoulder and said in a very gentle, controlled, and measured way, "Dad, don't we want to pray first?"

The enemy would have you believe all is lost. The enemy would have you believe that what you see is how it is going to be and that what you feel is real.

Our circumstances can bewilder us. The setbacks, the letdowns, the pain, the struggle—these can cause us to question whether there is a God at all and, if He is there, whether our struggle is beneath His power.

I believe in a big God with big plans and, as my friend and mentor Derek Grier says, a God who wants us to "live big"![3]

There is no big living when we are students of small thinking. I choose to see beyond the erosions in my hands, beyond the pain in my body, beyond the time that was lost, and beyond what life has cost and cling to the promises of God for my present and for my future!

So where am I today? The twenty-one days were the best days of my journey to discover how God cures. What started over twenty-five years ago, blossomed fifteen years ago, was used by the devil to try to kill me ten years ago, and Satan attempted to use to put the nails in the coffin five years ago has been met with my response—I am more than a conqueror. As Deuteronomy declares, "The LORD will make you the head and not the tail; you shall be above only, and not be beneath" (Deut. 28:13).

Take twenty-one days and venture to let God show you as He showed me. Put your soul on pause and connect your spirit to the will and purpose of God for your future. The gift in you is waiting, and the whole wide world will say, "Look what God has done."

Chapter 11

TWENTY-ONE DAYS TO DISCOVER THAT GOD CURES

GREW UP ABSOLUTELY hating the term *diet*. It was as if there was almost a battle between my grandmothers, as both seemingly were on diets my entire adolescence. Of course, as I became an adult, I grew to love the word, but for different reasons. I was as thin as a rail, but I worked in the industry of television direct-response infomercials as a writer and producer. Considering the more than thirty billion dollars spent each year on weight loss, I discovered that dieting was a national pastime.[1]

Research indicates that an estimated forty-five million Americans go on a diet each year.[2] While some fad diet is not often the answer for long-term weight loss, there are tremendous health benefits if someone drops as little as 5 percent of their total body weight. Studies show that we reduce the risk of osteo-arthritis, diabetes, stroke, and heart disease.[3]

And then there are the myriad autoimmune diseases that millions upon millions suffer with across the globe, and a condition that drove me with such passion to find how God cures. My Twenty-One-Day God Cures Diet (I'm now comfortable with the word) impacts autoimmune disease at its root.

WHY TWENTY-ONE DAYS?

I chose twenty-one days for a couple of reasons. First, it is a model set out by a fast entered into by the prophet Daniel.

> In those days I, Daniel, was mourning three full weeks. I ate no pleasant food, no meat or wine came into my mouth, nor did I anoint myself at all, till three whole weeks were fulfilled.
>
> —DANIEL 10:2–3

When you look at the results of the twenty-one-day fast, they were astonishing. I don't have space to detail it all here, but suffice it to say, they were significantly healthier than the others who were eating food that, quite candidly, resembles the standard American diet. The Twenty-One-Day God Cures Diet is *not* the Daniel fast. This is a comprehensive program designed to reveal to you the grand delusion and plan of Satan to kill, steal, and destroy your life, rob you of your future, erode your destiny, and blind you from ever discovering the gift and calling that God programmed in your DNA to be expressed in a positive way by your genes. Yeah, I said it. Let the really smart people begin the attack. I stand on the revelation that God gave me for you. Let's show the world what God can do when His children discover who He made them to be.

The second reason I chose twenty-one days is because I believe Daniel knew that it took twenty-one days to accomplish something. In the preface to *Psycho-Cybernetics* Dr. Maxwell Maltz wrote: "It usually requires a minimum of about 21 days to effect any perceptible change in a mental image. Following plastic surgery it takes about 21 days for the average patient to get used to his new face. When an arm or leg is amputated the 'phantom limb' persists for about 21 days. People must live in a new house for about three weeks before it begins to 'seem like home.' These, and many other commonly observed phenomena tend to show that it requires a minimum of about 21 days for an old mental image to dissolve and a new one to jell." [4]

Since Dr. Maltz published his book, people have used his twenty-one-day thing to pronounce that is how long it takes for habits to be formed or broken. Allow me to set the record straight that this period is not about it taking twenty-one days to create a habit. Many experts claim that this is nothing short of a myth.[5] If we're talking about habit formation, then let me be the one to tell you that it takes longer than that. This isn't about creating a habit; this is about cutting a God-made pattern of living. This is about change, and change from inside. This journey is about transformation, which is all about renewing your mind. I like the way the apostle Paul says it in Romans 12:2: "And do not be conformed to this world, but be transformed by the renewing of your mind, that you may prove what is that good and acceptable and perfect will of God."

For me, this journey was a process. I started week one with an intense fast from food that sent my entire world into orbit. I mean that in a positive sense. Is there something powerful about seven days? I don't know. I know that there was something powerful about committing to a time frame and sticking with it. This journey is all about commitment. But getting yourself eating right is only a diet unless you get your soul and spirit properly aligned. This is where the first seven days comes in: the fast. If you go on a diet and haven't changed the way you think, then what's going to happen when the diet ends? You got it. You will go right back to the way you lived before because you have not impacted the way you thought before.

You have a spirit, a soul, and a body. When you lead a soul-led life, the results are not good. But when you place your spirit at the top of our hierarchy, change happens. Getting in touch with God through prayer, worship, and reading the Bible revitalizes your spirit, giving it strength to lead the rest of your person. When you are led by your spirit, your soul starts behaving more like it should. Rather than reacting to things with anger and cynicism, you start displaying fruit of the Spirit, like kindness, gentleness, and self-control. When your spirit is healthy, your soul is going to be healthy.

The Twenty-One-Day God Cures Diet is a journey to total healing. I am not promoting discontinuing your prescribed medications (if you are on any), nor am I suggesting that you should cancel a scheduled doctor's visit or stop seeing your family practitioner. Thankfully, while much of this twenty-one-day plan was determined by trial and error across many years of starts and stops, failed attempts and ultimately success, I found several amazing alternative and natural wellness practitioners and non-conventional doctors who have pioneered this trail before me. They worked closely with me to fill in the holes that made this twenty-one-day plan complete.

DON'T EAT MEAT

This program is taking a bite out of the meat crime. We're going to completely restrict meat, as in don't eat any, for twenty-one days. Come on. You can do it!

You may be thinking, "I need protein." You will get it, naturally and toxin-free, from all the other great stuff you will be consuming on this program. And when you see the benefits of removing animals from your diet and the tremendous and almost miraculous benefits of a primarily plant-based diet, you will likely be eating less meat in a year than you used to consume in a month from your former life.

The World Health Organization has mounting evidence that processed meat consumption increases the risk of many types of disease, including cancer.[6] It is so profound that we should see labels on deli meats as we do on cigarettes. And meat is high in saturated fat. This is what can raise blood cholesterol. Remember, high levels of LDL cholesterol can increase the risk of heart disease. The industrialized meat industry rebukes this evidence and says there is no link between red meat and cancer and other diseases, as studies suggest. They claim that red meat fits perfectly into a diet that makes the body good.[7] But the truth is otherwise.

So why don't we know this? The problem is we are talking about billions of dollars at stake. Billions of dollars take the front seat, while your health and vitality take the back seat.

Organizations like the American Heart Association, American Arthritis Association, Diabetes Foundation, Susan G. Komen foundation, and other groups that promote finding cures and such are almost all taking money from the big food processing and packaging companies selling foodstuffs that are wreaking havoc in our bodies.[8] Hard to believe? Look it up on ZoeLogics .com. The hair will stand up on the back of your neck.

Remember the old saying, "You are what you eat"? It couldn't be more alarming, then, for you to discover the big meat corporations are feeding fish, pigs, sheep, chickens, and cattle pesticides (found in the grass and feed they are fed), antibiotics (injected into the animals and also infused into feed), steroids (the same), and even fecal matter.[9]

There are whistle-blowers coming out of the woodwork about industrialized meat plants that are packing toxic, decaying, rancid meatstuff but covering up the torrid and putrid smell with things like acid.[10] These packages end up sold to the public and even sold to schools to be fed to the future generation.

The principle for weight loss remains to burn more calories than you consume. This doesn't necessarily mean working out, although you will be exercising moderately with low-impact aerobics on this program. But your body will burn stored fat, which leads to rapid pound shedding when you substitute plant-based alternatives for the red and white stuff you've been eating.

Meat isn't good for you, at least not the meat we're getting today. Perhaps back in my grandfather's day, when they knew the chickens, pigs, and cows by name, things were different. Today it is nearly impossible to avoid toxicity when our consumption is of primarily processed and distressed meat products sold through our local grocery stores. I have listed a number of safe and reliable sources at ZoeLogics.com where you can get grass-fed meat, poultry without drugs pumped into them, and fresh, wild-caught fish.

DON'T EAT DAIRY

On the Twenty-One-Day God Cures Diet, it will be dairy no more. That means for twenty-one days absolutely no dairy. After twenty-one days, as with the meat, you will find that you will have very little interest in resuming your prior consumption levels of dairy.

And believe me, when I started out on the Twenty-One-Day God Cures Diet, I was a prolific eater, if you will, of dairy—a gallon of 2-percent milk a week, cheese, yogurt, creamer in my coffee. I absolutely loved dairy.

As does the world. The average American consumes two hundred and seventy-five pounds of dairy a year.[11] Wow. That is almost a pound a day. What does this translate into in terms of our health?

Well, the USDA (Department of Agriculture) recommends that we consume three cups of dairy products a day.[12] Wonder why? Because billions are at stake. Their recommendation is based on science barely strong enough to hold up in a court of law, if indeed the jury were comprised of nutritional experts that really understand how the body works.[13]

And this is how things go, generally speaking, across the board in the industrialized food world. You have major corporations that are in the business of making money off us, the consumers, pumping out all this propaganda about dietary needs so that we buy stuff that wrecks our bodies over time. And the corporations sponsor organizations that are searching for cures. A doctor friend of mine theorizes it is likely out of guilt.

But we are catching on. Studies indicate that dairy consumption is down 22 percent since 2005.[14] A switch to calcium-rich sources that impact bone health without side effects is on the rise—leafy greens (kale, spinach, collards, and broccoli, to name a few), tofu, or even those tasty little sardines (wild-caught of course). We can also fortify ourselves with a good vitamin D supplement. Look on my website, and you will see the one I take.

I dropped dairy and other animal products altogether, and I still enjoy the delicious foods I ate before but with alternatives such as almond milk, vegan pizza, and coconut milk. My body is thanking me for it.

Why? Simple. Almost two-thirds of humanity is lactose intolerant. This means that they lack an enzyme in their body that makes processing a protein in milk possible. The result? Digestive issues, inflammation, and more. Does that apply to you? An estimated 90 percent of East Asians, 80 percent of Central Asians (you never see cheese in an Asian restaurant), 80 percent of Native Americans, and 75 percent of African Americans are impacted.[15] For us Hebrews, no dairy. For my Latino friends, no more cheese. Or at least know that most of your digestive issues and inflammation are related. Research says consuming dairy when lactose intolerant leads to headaches/migraines, lethargy/fatigue, foggy mind, asthma, and skin problems (psoriasis/acne).[16]

My mother cut out dairy, and within twenty-one days she was asthma free, off her inhaler, and off steroids. The pharmaceutical industry hates us for this, and so do the insurance companies.

My son cut out dairy, and within thirty days he was off his medication too. His skin cleared up in weeks. I thank Kyle Craichy and his LXR-Organics for this revelation. You can see this entire study on my website.

No more dairy for twenty-one days. In twenty-one days, you will know what to do. You may reintroduce a small amount into your diet and then make a determination based upon how your body responds. For me, I have the smallest amount of cheese with some good wine one time per week. And when I tell you that I can tell, I wouldn't be exaggerating. I can feel the impact of dairy in a negative way almost instantly. Nevertheless, I am willing to push past the slight inconvenience. It's a personal choice. Balance.

BECOMING A PLANT-BASED EATER

This is going to be a culture shock for you if, like me, you have lived off the standard American diet your whole life. And when I tell you that you will have to walk out your healing because you've been on the American diet your whole life, it is no longer theory.

I want to encourage you that in twenty-one-days, you will see the benefits to continuing to remain primarily a plant-based eater. But for twenty-one-days it is rabbit food only!

Hopefully you didn't just quit on me. I know that this challenge seems like climbing Mount Everest. And at first, it might feel like it. I mean, you're going to have to muster some real courage and be prepared for some detox indicators (headache, low energy, immense cravings, etc.), but gradually you will begin to see the changes in your skin, your hair (if you have any), nails, waistline, digestion (no more constipation), and sleep, and you will never want to go back.

You are going to discover a love for beans, fruits, veggies, brown rice, potatoes, and other alternatives. Soon enough, when you see and feel the difference in your body, you won't want that other junk anymore that is designed to trigger what Satan wants—you to be slowed, restricted, and limited.

On my website, you will find some amazing recipes so you can learn how to cook stuff that you never thought could taste so good. And for those culinary experts, I am going to allow you to share your discoveries with this amazing new group of friends you will meet in the God Cures community. We can't wait to hear from you.

Here are the things that I recommend you do to get started. This is exactly what I did leading up to my Twenty-One-Day God Cures Diet, my journey to total and complete healing.

1. Purge the stuff that will tempt you.

Get in the cupboards and fridge and throw away everything that you won't be eating for the next twenty-one days. Don't give it to anyone. You don't want to contribute to Satan by helping him flip the epigenetics switch in anyone else.

Get your mind-set right. Most of the stuff you have in your cupboards and fridge isn't what God wants you to put in His temple. Most of that junk, while it's filling, is killing. Wait a minute, I need to tweet that: "It might be fillin', but it be killin'." Say that out loud as a declaration as you empty the pantry and fridge with a big trash bag. It will help do the trick to separate you from the stuff that your body doesn't need: refined sugar, candy, bread, eggs, meat of all types (including processed meat), soda, cooking oil, packaged crackers, packaged sweets, potato chips, milk, cheese, syrup, jelly, granola bars, boxed macaroni and cheese, and canned foods.

2. Get your family in alignment/agreement.

One of the most important things about your twenty-one-day journey to total healing is your support system. Don't try to be John Wayne or Wonder Woman or Dwayne "The Rock" Johnson and tough it through while everyone else around you is eating it up like the apocalypse is coming. It's the weirdest thing, but it seems that the moment you announce that you are going to fight Satan, suddenly everyone in your circumference ups the volume on junk that none of us should be eating. Get your support circle to get in agreement with what you are about to do. By agreement, I mean if they aren't joining you, then they will have the common courtesy of not bringing anything around you that you can't eat.

The concept of detoxing your body isn't about getting the foodstuff you've been gorging on for years out of your intestines.

And it is not just about your liver and kidneys doing the work and helping them along. It only takes forty-eight to seventy-two hours for your food to digest, so your body will get rid of what you have been carrying around in your gut naturally. After the initial fasting period (of at least two to three days, but seven days if you can muster it), when you start eating fresh fruits, vegetables, nuts, and seeds, you will be so regular that your body will cycle through what you put inside it within a twenty-four to thirty-six-hour period.

I want to make sure you understand that there is no balance or moderation in the twenty-one-day period. This is cold turkey. You aren't taking every sixth or seventh day off and getting a burger. I announced that I was drinking a latte and eating a burger at the opening of this book when I talked about no strict diets, but I wasn't referring to the twenty-one-day journey. Sorry. I was talking about after the journey.

During the twenty-one-days, we are driving the body to a place of restorative healing, down at a cellular level. This doesn't happen quickly, but it also doesn't take years. While some conditions that are more severe will require longer periods of time—perhaps a complete change of lifestyle and diet for months and months—what I am proposing can be accomplished in twenty-one-days.

So get your family and friends into alignment. We are only talking about twenty-one days. If they cannot support you for twenty-one-days, then we need to be having a different conversation about the people you have chosen to surround yourself with. I suggest that you give them *God Cures* to read for themselves.

One of the greatest ways to get your family into agreement with you on this journey is to invite them to the daily devotional. It is amazing how quickly we break through the soul-led barriers when we begin to invoke the life-giving, life-changing, and life-shifting Word of the living God.

> My soul clings to the dust; revive me according to Your word.
> —PSALM 119:25

3. Decide what day you will begin.

By now you have read the important chapters of the book. You are ready to get started. Getting started is all about planning. Planning incorporates many things, like number 1 and number 2, but also, it's about setting the right date to get started. If you are not one to plan, this one will be tough. I'm a pretty spontaneous person. I am a businessman, but more, I am an artist trapped in a businessman's body. Truth be known, I don't like to plan squat. I have to "feel" it. My grandfather used to tell me growing up that we cannot let our emotions be the determining factor as it pertains to whether or not we are going to do something. When it is time to get up to go to work, you can't let how you feel determine whether or not your feet hit the floor in the morning and get you going. You have to get going regardless of how you feel. Look to the heavens to motivate you. Colossians 3:2 says, "Set your mind on things above, not on things on the earth." This, in my view, is a great way to see things as we should see them. This journey is not about how you feel; this journey is about what God is trying to do in you and through you. So we are going to keep our eyes on Jesus, from whom our strength comes.

Nonetheless, you have to be practical. Planning is practical. Planning ensures that you don't get started next week, and a week later you're at some big wedding where the hors d'oeuvres, punch, and cake are going to cause you to fall off the wagon. Plan a starting point when you know your schedule is clear, you aren't traveling, and you don't have any big bar mitzvahs to go to.

SUPPRESSING THE SOUL THROUGH FASTING

There are so many fasts out there. Pastor Gregory Dickow has one (*From the Inside Out*—it's amazing); Cindy Trimm has one (*The 40-Day Soul Fast*—it's amazing); and Jentezen Franklin has one (*Fasting*—it's great too). There's the food fast, water-only fast, juice fast, carb fast, and Daniel fast. There's a forty-day fast, which my grandfather actually went on years ago; ten-day; twenty-one-day; and everything else in between.

Fasting works. Period. It is one of the most powerful physical disciplines, which wellness practitioners and medical doctors alike (if honest) report as having tremendous benefits for you and your body.

But fasting is also a tremendous spiritual discipline that God created and in fact called His prophets and apostles to, creating a supernatural method for them to enter into one of the most powerful pathways of focus, dialing into the Spirit of God and enabling them to receive insight, wisdom, knowledge, and deep spiritual things that only come through fasting and prayer. Let's certainly not forget that very important, necessary, and critical element: prayer.

You must prepare yourself for an all-out onslaught of attack from the enemy during your time of fasting. Let's face it, the last thing he wants is for you to suppress your soul man, giving a lift to your spirit man and allowing your spirit to get direction from the Almighty.

When I started my most recent fast, it was as if all hell broke loose. Fights erupted in my relationships, traffic on the road seemed more congested, and all my technology devices went haywire. What's more, Hurricane Harvey and Hurricane Irma hit us back to back within a matter of a few weeks. Our offices in Jacksonville, Florida, and Puerto Rico were devastated. Some might just say that this is all coincidence; however, I believe much of what happened in my personal and professional world was the enemy and his imps on high alert.

Expect and prepare to have new pressures, obstacles, and chaos at home, at work, at church, etc., that you didn't have before. But expecting it doesn't mean that you accept it. Just be ready for it, and by being ready for it, you will know how to respond to it.

How? Be patient. Respond in love. Know where your strength comes from. Know who's in control of the circumstances. Be slow to speak and quick to listen. Rest in Jesus and in the power of His might 24/7. Know that the weapons of your warfare aren't carnal but spiritual.

Every single one of those points is based upon what the Bible declares to be our response to adversity. So don't just be a reader of the Word; be a doer of it.

If you weren't a threat to the devil, he would leave you alone. Your declaration to fast is your declaration of taking ground from the enemy—taking your life back, subjecting it to the Lord, and casting out the schemes of Satan.

> By which have been given to us exceedingly great and pre-
> cious promises, that through these you may be partakers of
> the divine nature, having escaped the corruption that is in
> the world.
> —2 PETER 1:4

Regardless, when you do begin to incorporate real food back into your daily plan, I advise you to follow my do not eat and do eat lists below. I believe in moderation. I believe in balance. I do not believe in proposing that we stop living or enjoying the fruits of culinary discovery. I love chocolate cake. I just eat less now. Instead, my mind is disciplined, so I am no longer self-medicating by eating to fill the holes in my personality. I eat stuff I like because I enjoy it, and I control it, as opposed to it controlling me.

Within each day of your journey, here are the basics to keep in mind as it pertains to what to eat or what not to eat:

During the twenty-one-day journey, do not eat or drink:

- Sugar (Sugar is a destructive force that feeds disease, feeds inflammation, and will stand in the way of you getting well.)

- Diet sodas or any drinks of any kind that have aspartame or other artificial sweeteners

- Gluten (Do a Google search on foods with gluten and those without, and it will give you a pretty good sense of direction.)

- Dairy

- Meat

- Alcohol

- Fried foods

- Egg

- Corn oils, vegetable oils, and other cooking oils

And now the do (a lot) list:

- Drink eight to ten tall glasses of water every day for all twenty-one-days and the rest of your days! Stay away from bottled water. The plastic is loaded with chemicals, and there are a significant number of studies to prove it. Get a great water filter (see ZoeLogics.com) and hydrate, hydrate, hydrate. Put a slice of lemon in your glass too. It lowers your acidity and balances the pH levels in your body. Add a lime, and it's great for digestion and to diminish heartburn. Say good-bye to acid reducers.

- After the fast, eat lots of veggies (fresh and organic if you can afford it) like cauliflower, broccoli, kale, spinach, brussels sprouts, carrots, and cabbage.

- Consume a good B_{12} supplement every day and for the rest of your days. You can find some that I recommend on my website.

- Consume a good omega-3 supplement every day and for the rest of your days. See my website for recommendations.

- During and after the fast, eat fresh ginger, turmeric, cinnamon, rosemary, sage, and thyme.

- During and after the fast, eat coconut oil. Cook with it. Make a coffee shot with it (see the website).

- During and after the fast, eat olive oil (but not heated to high temperatures).

- After the fast, eat avocado, cucumbers, fermented foods (sauerkraut is my best friend), beans and legumes, nuts, and berries.

Disclaimer: It is OK to consult your doctor before beginning your fast. If you have severe or complicated health challenges that would cause you concern, then please modify your regimen based upon the advice of your health professional. Do not stop taking the medications prescribed by your health practitioner during the twenty-one-day journey.

The fast is comprised of more than just water. You may juice if you do not have my recommended meal shake. You can order your shakes on my website at ZoeLogics.com.

For the actual twenty-one-day plan, see the appendix. Each day has suggestions and tips to feed your body and your spirit while keeping all three parts of you in alignment.

CONCLUSION

S O, WHAT HAVE I learned?
I have learned that I am created in the image and likeness of a triune God. I am three parts; my soul possesses
a spirit, and they indwell my body, the temple of the Holy Spirit.

I have discovered that when sin entered the world, our spirit
died. At salvation, our spirit was made alive, and its intention is
to lead our life by being connected to the leading of God's Spirit.

I have discovered that our soul, a raging force, full of will and
emotion, is a weapon. Properly guided, which is to say, yielded to
our spirit, it is a force for the kingdom. Misguided, which would
be to say, getting its leading from the world, pop culture, entertainment, the government, higher education, the popular vote,
religion, our peers, etc., it can suppress the spirit, wreak havoc in
the world, wreck our lives, and destroy our bodies.

I have discovered a grand delusion, a diabolical plot of the
enemy to keep the gift planted inside of us from ever reaching

its place in the world, which would keep us from discovering our destiny, from living a life of purpose.

Satan knows the way the body works. He knows that buried in our physical structure, which is impacted by sin, humanity, now separated from the perfect garden, is subject to cellular decay and gene expression in this fallen world. He cannot control our minds, and he cannot win at war with us spiritually. He can, however, influence us by getting us to live a soul-led life. In so doing, Satan can nudge us in the wrong direction, which leads humanity on a path toward sickness, disease, and death, and in turn our life, our impact, and influence for the kingdom is cut short.

I have discovered that God has come that we might have life and have it abundantly—to the full (John 10:10). God can cure where the medical establishment cannot by healing me at the core of who I am. This is accomplished by discovering whose I am. This happens when I look to God, His Word, and His planned alignment for the triune part of me to become that which cures me.

As I center on Him, everything moves in proper order.

As I center on Him, I discover the valuable commodity that He gave me when He placed this soul, which possesses a spirit, into a body which would be the dwelling place of the Holy Spirit of God.

When I discover the value of my body, I realize the importance of caring for it, protecting it, and maintaining it.

I have discovered that God's Word is my source.

I have discovered that prayer is the greatest form of communication that I can engage in on earth.

I have discovered that I must eat well and eat right, and that my body will respond naturally.

I have discovered that God cures.

Appendix

TWENTY-ONE-DAY PLAN

SO HERE IS the plan. While the preferred period for the fast is three to seven days, just do your best. Remember that it is wise to consult your physician before starting the fast. Do not stop taking your prescribed medications without consulting a physician. Also, don't forget to get at least seven hours of sleep every night. Studies show that it is best to avoid eating anything after 8:00 p.m. so your food can be digested well before your head hits the pillow. And be sure to take the recommended B_{12} and omega-3 supplements (with the addition of a glutamine/glutathione supplement for those with severe autoimmune issues).

Make sure you drink eight to ten glasses of water a day. It is always a good idea to drink a glass of water with meals, and when you are studying the Word is another good time to sip a drink. Lemon water (room temperature water with a lemon slice) and warm tea (if you prefer cream, use almond milk or coconut milk; if you must have sweetener, use a tiny amount of organic honey) are good beverage choices.

Each day addresses topics such as meals, exercise, prayer, and studying the Word. There are suggestions for each meal, and recipes can be found on our website, but feel free to get creative with your fruits and veggies. There are scriptures suggested for your time studying the Word, as well as two passages to meditate on as you eat lunch and dinner. Spend time in prayer and meditation also considering how God's Word applies to you and your life. Prepare yourself, as the Word will begin to come alive to you! These things will feed your spirit.

DAY 1

Breakfast: Organic juice with flaxseed (for information on juicing, go to ZoeLogics.com) or SuperBerry or SuperGreens meal shake from LivingFuel; for those with severe autoimmune issues, substitute bone broth for a meal shake

Lunch: Organic juice with flaxseed or bone broth

Dinner: Meal shake or bone broth

Verses for prayer and meditation: Romans 4

"For I will restore health to you and heal you of your wounds," says the LORD.

—JEREMIAH 30:17

Oh restore me to health and make me live!

—ISAIAH 38:16, ESV

Exercise: If you live in a safe neighborhood, try thirty minutes of brisk walking. If you have a treadmill, start treading. Some people find vacuuming or cleaning the house a good workout. The bottom line here is to get mobile and get the heart pumping. Be sure to stretch first, and remember to stay hydrated!

DAY 2

Breakfast: Organic juice with flaxseed or SuperBerry or SuperGreens meal shake from LivingFuel; for those with severe autoimmune issues, substitute bone broth for a meal shake

Lunch: Organic juice with flaxseed or bone broth

Dinner: Meal shake or bone broth

Verses for prayer and meditation: Romans 5

Then your light shall break forth like the morning, your healing shall spring forth speedily, and your righteousness shall go before you; the glory of the LORD shall be your rear guard.

—ISAIAH 58:8

But for you who fear my name, the sun of righteousness shall rise with healing in its wings. You shall go out leaping like calves from the stall.

—MALACHI 4:2, ESV

Exercise: Kick it up a notch and head to your local gym. Find an exercise or apparatus that matches your level of fitness. An elliptical workout is always a good choice. Remember to stretch before and after working out!

DAY 3

Breakfast: Organic juice with flaxseed or SuperBerry or SuperGreens meal shake from LivingFuel; for those with severe autoimmune issues, substitute bone broth for a meal shake

Lunch: Organic juice with flaxseed or bone broth

Dinner: Meal shake or bone broth

Verses for prayer and meditation: Romans 6

But He was wounded for our transgressions, He was bruised for our iniquities; the chastisement for our peace was upon Him, and by His stripes we are healed.

—Isaiah 53:5

Heal me, O Lord, and I shall be healed; save me, and I shall be saved, for You are my praise.

—Jeremiah 17:14

Exercise: Think of something enjoyable to do for exercise today. You could jump rope, play basketball, go bike riding, or even play tennis. Find an activity you enjoy doing and get family and friends involved as well. The more you enjoy exercising, the more you will stick with it.

Congratulations! You made it through three full days of fasting. The first three days you may have experienced some of the detox indicators I mentioned earlier (headache, low energy, immense cravings, etc.). But be encouraged—you will gradually begin to see positive changes in your body. I encourage those who can to continue on liquid and meal shakes only for the next four days. However, for the others, you can start eating fresh fruits, vegetables, nuts, and seeds (organic is preferred).

Day 4

≈

Breakfast: Organic juice with flaxseed or SuperBerry or SuperGreens meal shake from LivingFuel; for those with severe autoimmune issues, substitute bone broth for a meal shake. Or eat some fruit with your shake.

Lunch: Organic juice with flaxseed or bone broth; or fresh vegetables, such as a spinach and kale salad with fresh fruit and nuts

Dinner: Meal shake or bone broth; or vegetable salad or vegetable plate

Verses for prayer and meditation: Romans 7–8

Come to Me, all you who labor and are heavy laden, and I will give you rest. Take My yoke upon you and learn from Me, for I am gentle and lowly in heart, and you will find rest for your souls. For My yoke is easy and My burden is light.

—MATTHEW 11:28–30

In Him we have redemption through His blood, the forgiveness of sins, according to the riches of His grace.

—EPHESIANS 1:7

Exercise: If you do not have a gym membership or cannot get to a gym, let me suggest going to the park today. You can go for a brisk walk, jog, jump rope, and even do some push-ups or sit-ups.

Day 5

Breakfast: Organic juice with flaxseed or
SuperBerry or SuperGreens meal shake from
LivingFuel; for those with severe autoimmune
issues, substitute bone broth for a meal shake. Or
eat some fruit with your shake.

Lunch: Organic juice with flaxseed or bone
broth; or fresh vegetables, such as a green leafy
salad with fresh fruit and nuts

Dinner: Meal shake or bone broth; or fresh leafy
salad or vegetable plate with some fresh fruit
and nuts

Verses for prayer and meditation: Romans 12

The LORD will keep you free from every disease. He will
not inflict on you the horrible diseases you knew in Egypt.
—DEUTERONOMY 7:15, NIV

Now faith is the substance of things hoped for, the evidence
of things not seen.
—HEBREWS 11:1

Exercise: Consider doing an exercise you have
never done before. I tried yoga, and now I am a
big fan. You may want to try it out. I found it to
be a great activity to partner with my spiritual

exercises, such as meditation of Scripture. It also helps with stretching and flexibility.

Day 6

Breakfast: Organic juice with flaxseed or SuperBerry or SuperGreens meal shake from LivingFuel; for those with severe autoimmune issues, substitute bone broth for a meal shake. Or eat some fruit with your shake.

Lunch: Organic juice with flaxseed or bone broth; or spinach salad with fresh fruit, nuts, and carrots

Dinner: Meal shake or bone broth; or fresh green leafy salad or vegetable plate with fresh fruit and nuts

Verses for prayer and meditation: Ephesians 1

Blessed are those who have regard for the weak; the LORD delivers them in times of trouble. The LORD protects and preserves them—they are counted among the blessed in the land—he does not give them over to the desire of their foes. The LORD sustains them on their sickbed and restores them from their bed of illness.

—PSALM 41:1–3, NIV

I will praise the LORD according to His righteousness, and will sing praise to the name of the LORD Most High.

—PSALM 7:17

Exercise: If you have access to a swimming pool, try swimming today (outdoors if the weather is good). The natural buoyancy of being in the water makes movement much easier on your joints. This is also a great way to work out some of your muscles. If you do not have access to a pool, then try going for a walk.

DAY 7

Breakfast: Organic juice with flaxseed or SuperBerry or SuperGreens meal shake from LivingFuel; for those with severe autoimmune issues, substitute bone broth for a meal shake. Or eat some fruit with your shake.

Lunch: Organic juice with flaxseed or bone broth; or spinach salad with fresh fruit, nuts, and carrots

Dinner: Meal shake or bone broth; or fresh spinach and kale salad or vegetable plate with fresh fruit and nuts

Verses for prayer and meditation: Ephesians 2

Beloved, I pray that you may prosper in all things and be in health, just as your soul prospers.

—3 JOHN 1:2

I will greatly rejoice in the LORD, my soul shall be joyful in my God; for He has clothed me with the garments of salvation, He has covered me with the robe of righteousness.

—ISAIAH 61:10

> **Exercise:** Now that you have spent the past several days exercising in different and unique ways, I want you to exercise today in whichever way you liked the most. If you can find a way to make exercising enjoyable, you will do it more often and stay consistent with it.

Congratulations! You made it through seven days of fasting—not an easy feat! Look into the mirror, and give yourself some affirmation. Give verbal affirmation to yourself that you like who you are and the way you look.

Hopefully before you began the journey, you planned and prepared by doing a little shopping in the organic section of your local grocery store or shopping online at a source for organic foods. I highly recommend that if you haven't stocked for the next fourteen days, you make it part of what you do first thing this morning or on your lunch break. If you have been fasting the entire seven days, by now you are really hungry; if you wait too long to get to the store you're going to be susceptible to cheating. The plan will contain several ideas for each meal (you can find recipes on ZoeLogics.com). Find one you like or come up with your own ideas that incorporate leafy green vegetables, fresh fruit, nuts, seeds, beans, legumes, and whole grains.

DAY 8

Breakfast: Steel Cut Oatmeal With Favorite Fruit and Nuts; Kale and Sweet Potato Pancakes; Shredded Wheat Cereal With Plant Milk (Almond or Coconut) and Favorite Fruit; or Tofu Scramble With Sweet Potato

Lunch: Plant Protein Packed Peppers; Spinach and Kale Salad With Strawberries and Nuts; Cucumber Salad; Sweet Potato and Black Bean Soup; Cauliflower Purée Soup; or Veggie Burger

Dinner: Eggplant Rotolo; Mushroom Lasagna; Lentil Butternut Squash Shepherd's Pie; Mushroom Soup; Cabbage Soup; Boston Chard Salad; or Apple Salad With Mint and Pine Nuts

Verses for prayer and meditation: Ephesians 3

Your words were found, and I ate them, and Your word was to me the joy and rejoicing of my heart; for I am called by Your name, O LORD God of hosts.

—JEREMIAH 15:16

Bless the LORD, O my soul, and forget not all His benefits: who forgives all your iniquities, who heals all your diseases, who redeems your life from destruction, who crowns you with lovingkindness and tender mercies.

—PSALM 103:2–4

Exercise: If the weather permits, go to the park today. Take a brisk walk, taking time to reflect and appreciate God's creation in nature. God can speak to us through nature, but we don't always take time to look for Him or wait to hear from Him in this manner. If you cannot get outside, then jump rope, run in place, vacuum, or clean up in close proximity to a window so you can still seek God in nature.

DAY 9

Breakfast: Bob's Red Mill High Fiber Cereal; Cold Muesli (you can add blueberries, strawberries, or bananas); Zucchini Bread; or Apple Cinnamon Breakfast Parfait

Lunch: Curried Butternut Squash Soup; Kale Salad With Eggplant; Chipotle Hummus Wrap; Vegetable Tacos; Vegan Caesar Salad; Raw Beet Salad; Kale and White Bean Soup; or Bean Stew With Parsnip Mash

Dinner: Kidney Bean and Yam Soup; Black Bean Chili; Hearty Vegetable Stew; Zucchini With Onion, Tomato, and Mushrooms; Brown Rice and Vegetables; Quinoa With Oven Sautéed Mushrooms; or Lentil Burger With Baked Sweet Potato

Verses for prayer and meditation: Ephesians 4

For I know the plans I have for you, declares the LORD, plans for welfare and not for evil, to give you a future and a hope.

—JEREMIAH 29:11, ESV

Surely there is a future, and your hope will not be cut off.

—PROVERBS 23:18, ESV

Exercise: If the weather permits and you have a bike, ride around your neighborhood this morning. If you do not own a bike, then run or jog around your neighborhood. If you cannot get outside, then pick up some weights and pump some iron.

DAY 10

Breakfast: Banana Pinwheels; Vegan Sausage and Apple Breakfast; Watermelon Rolls; or Baked Steel Cut Oatmeal

Lunch: Quinoa Zucchini Burgers; Mango Gazpacho; Radish Sandwich With Arugula; Orzo Spinach Soup; White Bean and Millet Soup; or Salad Wraps With Beans and Greens

Dinner: Squash and Garbanzo Curry; Vegan Mongolian Beef With Broccoli; Stewed Zucchini With Basil and Mint; Baby Bok Choy and

Vegetable Stir Fry; Baked Vegan Enchiladas; or
Fresh Lentil Salad With Cherry Tomatoes

Verses for prayer and meditation: Ephesians 5

Or do you not know that your body is the temple of the
Holy Spirit who is in you, whom you have from God, and
you are not your own? For you were bought at a price; therefore glorify God in your body and in your spirit, which
are God's.

—1 CORINTHIANS 6:19–20

If then your whole body is full of light, having no part dark,
the whole body will be full of light, as when the bright
shining of a lamp gives you light.

—LUKE 11:36

Exercise: Let's change it up a little and lift some
weights today. Go to the gym, pump some iron,
or maybe take a class they may be offering.
You should be feeling good with lots of energy
to burn.

DAY 11

Breakfast: Bell Pepper Breakfast Burrito; Peach
Apple Blueberry Chaat; Strawberry Lemon
Lavender Muffins; or Blueberry Pomegranate
Smoothie

Lunch: Mashed Plantain With Red Beans; Sweet Potato Frittata; Butternut Squash Apple Burgers; Braised Cabbage Rolls; Ginger Orzo Brussels Sprouts Salad; or Autumn Vegetable Curry

Dinner: Lentil Nut Loaf With Sweet Potato; Grilled Tofu and Vegetable Shish Kebabs; Red Quinoa Enchiladas Rojas; Black Bean Quinoa Mango Medley; Brown Rice Risotto With Caramelized Onions, Squash, and Broccoli; or Grilled Wild Caught Salmon With Asparagus and Cauliflower Mashed Potatoes

Verses for prayer and meditation: Philippians 2

Your word is a lamp to my feet and a light to my path.
—PSALM 119:105

Be anxious for nothing, but in everything by prayer and supplication, with thanksgiving, let your requests be made known to God; and the peace of God, which surpasses all understanding, will guard your hearts and minds through Christ Jesus.
—PHILIPPIANS 4:6–7

Exercise: Let's mix it up again today. Run in place for a minute, rest for thirty seconds, do squats for a minute, rest for thirty seconds, do jumping jacks for a minute, and rest for a full minute. Repeat two more times. Rest for a full two minutes. Then do push-ups for a minute, rest for thirty seconds, do sit-ups for a minute, rest for thirty seconds, do burpees for a minute, and rest for a full minute. Repeat two more times. You should be tired but feeling great!

Day 12

Breakfast: Spinach and Kale Smoothie With Fresh Berries and Seeds; Berry Breakfast Couscous; Maple Date Pumpkin Porridge; or Chocolate Avocado Smoothie

Lunch: Artichoke Spinach Strata; Cabbage and Carrot Crunch Salad; Sweet Peanut Burgers; Zucchini Noodles; Lentil Burger; or Veggie Wrap (avocado, tomatoes, lettuce, and onion)

Dinner: Lentil Baked Potato Curry Patties; Brown Rice Stuffed Carnival Squash; Cavolo Nero: Kale and White Bean Soup; Shiitake Onion Miso Soup; Boston Romaine Salad; or Moroccan Pumpkin Stew

Verses for prayer and meditation: Philippians 3

My son, give attention to my words; incline your ear to my sayings. Do not let them depart from your eyes; keep them in the midst of your heart; for they are life to those who find them, and health to all their flesh.

—Proverbs 4:20–22

Let the words of my mouth and the meditation of my heart be acceptable in your sight, O LORD, my strength and my Redeemer.

—PSALM 19:14

Exercise: Jump on the treadmill or elliptical today for a good cardio workout. Listen to some upbeat Christian music as you work out today.

DAY 13

⌒

Breakfast: Coconut Raisin Flax Granola; Blueberry Lassi (Smoothie); or Rice Pudding With Berries

Lunch: Baked Rosemary Mushroom Polenta; Blood Orange Fennel Salad; Roasted Delicata Squash Boats; Walnut Almond Lettuce Wraps; Mini Mushroom Burgers; or Tahini Quinoa Bean Salad

Dinner: Brown Rice and Beans; Stuffed Acorn Squash; Red Lentil Chili in an Acorn Squash; Tri-Color Quinoa Salad; Chana Masala Kale Bowl; Kale, Sweet Potato, and Carrot Curry; or Spinach and Artichoke Lasagna

Verses for prayer and meditation: Philippians 4

God is our refuge and strength, a very present help in trouble. Therefore we will not fear, even though the earth be removed, and though the mountains be carried into the midst of the sea; though its waters roar and be troubled, though the mountains shake with its swelling.

—PSALM 46:1–3

Show me Your ways, O LORD; teach me Your paths. Lead me in Your truth and teach me, for You are the God of my salvation; on You I wait all the day.

—PSALM 25:4–5

Exercise: Stretching is so important that I have decided it will be the exercise of the day. You may consider yoga this morning. While you are stretching, play some soft, soothing Christian music in the background. Focus on your breathing while you are stretching. Be sure to breathe in through your nose and out through your mouth as you engage your muscles while stretching.

DAY 14

Breakfast: Chocolate Almond Smoothie; Breakfast Chili; Polenta Breakfast With Dried Fruits and Nuts; or Turmeric Scrambled Tofu

Lunch: Curried Butternut Velvet Soup; Chilled Beet Soup With Dill Croutons; Asian Tofu Wraps; Eggplant Tempeh Bolognese Napoleon; Lentil Burger; or Spicy Grapefruit and Jicama Spinach Salad

Dinner: Smashed Olive Pasta/Quinoa;
Mediterranean Vegetable Noodle Soup; Burritos
(hummus, black beans, brown rice, and spinach);
Grilled Eggplant Sandwich With Baked Potato
Fries; Hopi Vegetable Stew; Escalivada (Catalan
Roast Vegetables); or Vegan Huevos Rancheros
Casserole

Verses for prayer and meditation: John 1

Death and life are in the power of the tongue, and those
who love it will eat its fruit.

—PROVERBS 18:21

My mouth shall speak wisdom, and the meditation of my
heart shall give understanding.

—PSALM 49:3

Exercise: If the weather permits, go to the
park and enjoy a brisk walk. You can also walk
around your neighborhood. You may even
want to jog a little to get the heart pumping.
Otherwise, you can stay in, lift some weights,
and jump rope.

DAY 15

Breakfast: Apple-Date Crockpot Cereal;
Raspberry Peach Blender Breakfast Smoothie;
Stewed Oats With Berries; or Breakfast
Melon Bowl

Lunch: Cree Bean Salad; Broccoli Mandarin Orange Salad; Broccoli, Red Pepper, and Tofu Quiche; Spanish Couscous Salad; Black Beans and Rice; or Grilled Veggie Sandwich

Dinner: Broccoli Burritos; Jackfruit Krabby Patty; Spicy Black Beans and Greens Over Brown Rice; Swiss Chard and Rice Balls Over Brown Rice; Cauliflower Mashed Potatoes With Mixed Vegetables; Black-Eyed Peas and Bitter Greens Casserole; or Three-Bean Chili Over Brown Rice

Verses for prayer and meditation: John 3

For You formed my inward parts; You covered me in my mother's womb. I will praise You, for I am fearfully and wonderfully made; marvelous are Your works, and that my soul knows very well.

—Psalm 139:13–14

My frame was not hidden from You, when I was made in secret, and skillfully wrought in the lowest parts of the earth. Your eyes saw my substance, being yet unformed. And in Your book they all were written, the days fashioned for me, when as yet there were none of them. How precious also are Your thoughts to me, O God! How great is the sum of them!

—Psalm 139:15–17

Exercise: Pick the exercise that you enjoy doing the most. Don't make it too easy, but enjoy yourself. You may even decide to play some music during your workout time.

DAY 16

Breakfast: Mushroom Frittata; Eggplant Bell Pepper Kugel; Blue Brainiac Smoothie; or Steel Cut Oatmeal With Blueberries

Lunch: Carrot Soup With Parsnip Ships; Cucumber Salad; Mexican Tofu Scramble; Grilled Onion Eggplant Sandwiches; Grilled Pineapple Watermelon Salad; or Spanish Marinated Portobello Mushrooms

Dinner: Sheet Pan Ratatouille With Creamy Polenta; Black-Eyed Pea Chili; Garlic-Rosemary Broccoli and Mushrooms With Brown Rice; Warm Lentil Salad; Chickpea Quinoa Burger; Stuffed Mushrooms Over Broccoli Cauliflower Mashed Potatoes; or Wild Caught Salmon Over Brown Rice With Broccoli

Verses for prayer and meditation: John 6

If one of your brethren becomes poor, and falls into poverty among you, then you shall help him, like a stranger or a sojourner, that he may live with you.

—LEVITICUS 25:35

Therefore, as the elect of God, holy and beloved, put on tender mercies, kindness, humility, meekness, longsuffering; bearing with one another, and forgiving one another, if

anyone has a complaint against another; even as Christ for-
gave you, so you also must do.

—COLOSSIANS 3:12–13

Exercise: Go bike riding this morning if the
weather permits. If not, head to the gym and
swim a few laps in the pool. This will relax you
but also strengthen and elongate your muscles.
Getting on the treadmill is another good option
for exercise today.

DAY 17

Breakfast: Crustless Broccoli Sun-Dried Tomato
Quiche; Mint Chocolate Smoothie; Whole Grain
Muesli; or Blueberry Lemon Bars

Lunch: Black Bean Burger; Whole Grain Pasta
Primavera; Mushroom, Onion, and Spinach
Stuffed Peppers; Vegan Chiles Rellenos;
Mushroom Stroganoff; or Quinoa Salad With
Spinach

Dinner: Sweet Potato Vegetable Lasagna; Black
Bean Beet Burger With Baked Sweet Potato
Fries; Stuffed Poblano Chiles With Pineapple
Salsa; Eggplant Szechuan Style With Peppers
and Mushrooms; Vegetarian Chili; Broccoli
Cauliflower Veggie Divan; or One-Pot Penne
Pasta With Tomato Cream Sauce

Verses for prayer and meditation: John 8

Make a joyful shout to the LORD, all you lands! Serve the LORD with gladness; come before His presence with singing. Know that the LORD, He is God; it is He who has made us, and not we ourselves; we are His people and the sheep of His pasture.

—PSALM 100:1–3

Enter into His gates with thanksgiving, and into His courts with praise. Be thankful to Him, and bless His name. For the LORD is good; His mercy is everlasting, and His truth endures to all generations.

—PSALM 100:4–5

Exercise: Let's go back to something you did earlier. Run in place for a minute, rest for thirty seconds, do squats for a minute, rest for thirty seconds, do jumping jacks for a minute, and rest for a full minute. Repeat two more times. Rest for a full two minutes. Then do push-ups for a minute, rest for thirty seconds, do sit-ups for a minute, rest for thirty seconds, do burpees for a minute, and rest for a full minute. Repeat two more times.

DAY 18

Breakfast: Chickpea Cauliflower Quiche; Maple and Curry Roasted Walnuts; Oil-Free Buckwheat

Crackers With Sunflower Seeds; or Peach Vanilla
Smoothie

Lunch: Butternut Squash Pasta With Sage
Mushrooms; Black Bean Meatless Balls and
Zucchini Noodles; Thai Potato Ginger Curry;
Root Vegetable Samosas; Curried Tofu "Egg"
Salad With Almonds; or Black-Eyed Pea Salad

Dinner: Spaghetti Squash Noodles With Spicy
Peanut Sauce; Veggie Lo Mein; Lotsa Green
Lasagna; Zesty Papaya Salad; Corn and Black
Bean Burritos; Hearty Tomato-Eggplant Pasta; or
Cauliflower and Chickpea Curry

Verses for prayer and meditation: John 9

But if we hope for what we do not see, we eagerly wait for
it with perseverance.... And we know that all things work
together for good to those who love God, to those who are
the called according to His purpose.
—ROMANS 8:25, 28

We...do not cease to pray for you, and to ask that you may
be filled with the knowledge of His will in all wisdom and
spiritual understanding; that you may walk worthy of the
Lord, fully pleasing Him, being fruitful in every good work
and increasing in the knowledge of God; strengthened with
all might, according to His glorious power, for all patience
and longsuffering with joy.
—COLOSSIANS 1:9–11

Exercise: Let's focus on strength training today.
Do thirty jumping jacks, ten push-ups, ten to

twenty squats, and ten to twenty front lunges. Rest, and then do it again three more times. This should really get you moving.

DAY 19

Breakfast: Watermelon Gazpacho; Breakfast Chili; Ginger Peach Crumble; or Peach Apple Blueberry Chaat

Lunch: Italian White Beans With Kale; French Lentil Salad With Cherry Tomatoes; Spinach and Raspberry Salad; Apricot Cilantro Quinoa Pilaf; Sweet Potato Chili Over Couscous; or Spinach Black Bean Burritos

Dinner: Meatless Meatloaf; Vegetable Minestrone; Antipasto Salad With Potatoes; Spinach Corn Enchiladas; Yellow Squash Chili; Sautéed Artichokes in Lemon; or Maple Sweet Potato Ravioli

Verses for prayer and meditation: John 10

Mercy and truth have met together; righteousness and peace have kissed.

—PSALM 85:10

When a man's ways please the LORD, He makes even his enemies to be at peace with him.

—PROVERBS 16:7

Exercise: This is a good day for stretching. Do yoga or some other stretching activity that will loosen and lengthen your muscles. It's important to remember to breathe in through your nose and out from your mouth as you stretch your muscles.

DAY 20

⁀

Breakfast: Shredded Wheat Cereal With Almond or Coconut Milk (add your favorite fruit); Cold Muesli (add blueberries, strawberries, or bananas); Steel Cut Oatmeal (add your favorite fruit and nuts); or Kale and Sweet Potato Pancakes

Lunch: Spicy Grapefruit and Jicama Spinach Salad; Quesadillas Zucchini Style; Tomato-Zucchini Bake; Sautéed Moroccan Butternut Squash; Wild Rice Black-Eyed Pea Patties; or Zesty Bean Gumbo

Dinner: Beet, Pear, and Endive Salad; Brûléed Squash With Pepitos; Maitake Squash Blossom Fettuccine; Portobello Mushroom Burgers; Mushroom Wellington; Eggplant Zucchini Bean Loaf; or Pasta e Fagioli

Verses for prayer and meditation: John 12

But those who wait on the LORD shall renew their strength; they shall mount up with wings like eagles, they shall run and not be weary, they shall walk and not faint.

—ISAIAH 40:31

And let us not grow weary while doing good, for in due season we shall reap if we do not lose heart.

—GALATIANS 6:9

Exercise: Feel free to do whatever you feel like doing at the gym today. You could go swimming or get on the elliptical or treadmill. You could even lift weights. Your fitness activity today is completely up to you to decide.

DAY 21

Breakfast: Watermelon Rolls; Steel Cut Oatmeal With Fruit; Blueberry Pomegranate Smoothie; or Berry Breakfast Couscous

Lunch: Cranberry Almond Stuffed Squash; White Bean and Millet Soup; Salad Wraps With Beans and Greens; Sweet Potato Frittata; Butternut Squash Apple Burgers; or Veggie Wrap (avocado, tomatoes, lettuce, and onion)

Dinner: Vegan Mongolian Beef With Broccoli; Stewed Zucchini With Basil and Mint; Mashed Plantain With Red Beans; Brown Rice Risotto With Caramelized Onions, Squash, and Broccoli;

Grilled Wild-Caught Salmon With Asparagus
and Cauliflower Mashed Potatoes; Lentil Baked
Potato Curry Patties; or Spinach and Artichoke
Lasagna

Verses for prayer and meditation: John 15

But without faith it is impossible to please Him, for he who
comes to God must believe that He is, and that He is a
rewarder of those who diligently seek Him.

—HEBREWS 11:6

Giving all diligence, add to your faith virtue, to virtue
knowledge, to knowledge self-control, to self-control perseverance, to perseverance godliness, to godliness brotherly
kindness, and to brotherly kindness love.

—2 PETER 1:5–7

Exercise: Freely choose your favorite exercise
for today. Whatever you feel like doing, do it,
but make it count. Give all you have, and hold
nothing back. Crank the music up today if you
can and celebrate your accomplishment.

If you go online to ZoeLogics.com, you can print out this entire
twenty-one-day regimen. All you have to do is print it and follow
it as I followed it. On the website I also have other resources and
valuable information available to you! I am proud of you, and
I'm rooting for you!

NOTES

PREFACE

1. *Merriam-Webster*, s.v. "limited," accessed September 19, 2017, https://www.merriam-webster.com/dictionary/limited.
2. "FAQs," *Defense POW/MIA Accounting Agency*, accessed September 19, 2017, http://www.dpaa.mil/Resources/FAQs/; "Fiscal Year 2017 President's Budget Defense POW/MIA Accounting Agency (DPAA)," *US Department of Defense*, February 2016, http://comptroller.defense.gov/Portals/45/Documents/defbudget/FY2017/budget_justification/pdfs/01_Operation_and_Maintenance/O_M_VOL_1_PART_1/DPAA_OP-5.pdf.

INTRODUCTION

1. "Hippocrates," *Wikipedia,* last updated September 25, 2017, https://en.wikipedia.org/wiki/Hippocrates.

2. A. R. Bernard, *Happiness Is...: Simple Steps to a Life of Joy* (New York: Simon and Schuster, 2006), vii, https://books.google .com/books?id=VikY_vaFXVUC&q.

3. Joel D. Wallach, *Dead Doctors Don't Lie* (Bonita, CA: Wellness Publications LLC, 1999).

4. "Dikembe Mutombo," *Wikipedia,* last updated September 17, 2017, https://en.wikipedia.org/wiki/Dikembe_Mutombo.

CHAPTER 1
LOOKING FOR ANSWERS

1. Oswald Chambers, "Do You See Jesus in Your Clouds?," *My Utmost for His Highest,* July 29, updated version, https://utmost .org/do-you-see-jesus-in-your-clouds/.

CHAPTER 2
HEALED OR CURED?

1. "Global Health Observatory Data, Health Workforce, Aggregated Data, Absolute Numbers," *World Health Organization*, updated February 7, 2017, http://apps.who.int/gho/data /node.main.A1443?lang=en&showonly=HWF.

2. Stephanie Bucklin, "8 Mammals That Have Been Cloned Since Dolly the Sheep," *Live Science*, February 22, 2017, https:// www.livescience.com/57971-mammals-that-have-been-cloned .html; Mindy Weisberger, "11 Body Parts Grown in the Lab," *Live Science*, July 3, 2017, https://www.livescience.com/59675 -body-parts-grown-in-lab.html.

3. Tyger Latham, "Mental Illness on the Rise in the U.S.," *Psychology Today*, May 18, 2011, https://www.psychologytoday .com/blog/therapy-matters/201105/mental-illness-the-rise-in -the-us.

4. *Merriam-Webster,* s.v. "epi-," accessed October 2, 2017, https://www.merriam-webster.com/dictionary/epi-.

5. "Gene," *Wikipedia,* last updated September 16, 2017, https://en.wikipedia.org/wiki/Gene.

6. "How Are New DNA Molecules Made?," J. Craig Venter Institute, updated January 15, 2003, http://www.genomenews network.org/resources/whats_a_genome/Chp1_4_2.shtml.

7. Angela L. Duker, "The Basics on Genes and Genetic Disorders," *The Nemours Foundation*, June 2013, http://m.kidshealth.org /en/teens/genes-genetic-disorders.html.

8. Duker, "The Basics on Genes and Genetic Disorders."

9. Vocabulary.com, s.v. "symptomatic," accessed October 9, 2017, https://www.vocabulary.com/dictionary/symptomatic.

10. Douglas Main, "95 Percent of People Have Some Illness or Injury," *Newsweek*, June 10, 2015, accessed October 4, 2017, http://www.newsweek.com/95-percent-people-have-some -illness-or-injury-341473.

11. Main, "95 Percent of People Have Some Illness or Injury."

12. Norene Anderson, "10 Most Common Health Diseases," LiveStrong.com, updated August 14, 2017, http://www .livestrong.com/article/161780-10-most-common-health -diseases/.

13. Barry L. Beyerstein, "Do We Really Use Only 10 Percent of Our Brains?," *Scientific American*, accessed October 2, 2017, https://www.scientificamerican.com/article/do-we-really-use-only-10/.

14. "True or False: An Apple a Day Keeps the Doctor Away," *Aspen Family Medicine at Green Valley Ranch*, EBSCO Publishing, accessed October 2, 2017, https://aspenfamilymed.secure.ehc .com/hl/?/156968/True-or-False--An-Apple-a-Day-Keeps-the -Doctor-Away; Lauren Steussy, "5 Ways Sugar Could Kill You," *New York Post*, January 11, 2017, http://nypost.com /2017/01/11/5-ways-sugar-could-kill-you/.

15. Jacque Wilson, "Are Bananas Bad for Me, Too?," *Cable News Network*, January 15, 2014, http://www.cnn.com/2014/01/15 /health/bananas-nutritional-benefits/index.html.

16. Hannah Nichols, "Dairy: Is It Good or Bad for You?," *Medical News Today*, June 19, 2017, https://www.medicalnewstoday.com /articles/317993.php.

17. "Butter vs. Margarine," *Harvard University Health Publishing*, accessed October 2, 2017, https://www.health.harvard.edu /nutrition/butter-vs-margarine.

18. Daniel Lieber, Kerry Samerotte, and Brian Beliveau, "You Are What Your Mother Ate: The Science of Epigenetics," *Science in the News*, Harvard Medical School lecture, October 6, 2010, accessed October 4, 2017, http://sitn.hms.harvard.edu/wp -content/uploads/2010/09/Epigenetics-Part-1.pdf.

19. Lieber, Samerotte, and Beliveau, "You Are What Your Mother Ate."

CHAPTER 3
THE GRAND DELUSION

1. *Merriam-Webster*, s.v. "cure," accessed September 27, 2017, https://www.merriam-webster.com/dictionary/cure.

2. *Blue Letter Bible*, s.v. "*satan*," accessed September 27, 2017, https://www.blueletterbible.org/lang/lexicon/lexicon.cfm ?Strongs=H7854&t=KJV.

3. *Oxford English Dictionary*, s.v. "iniquity," accessed September 27, 2017, https://en.oxforddictionaries.com/definition/iniquity.

4. *Merriam-Webster*, s.v. "cell," accessed September 27, 2017, https://www.merriam-webster.com/dictionary/cell.

5. James Gallagher, "'Memories' Pass Between Generations," *BBC*, December 1, 2013, http://www.bbc.com/news/health-25156510.

6. Lieber, Samerotte, and Beliveau, "You Are What Your Mother Ate."

7. Dan Hurley, "Grandma's Experiences Leave a Mark on Your Genes," *Discover*, May 2013, accessed October 4, 2017, http://discovermagazine.com/2013/may/13-grandmas-experiences-leave-epigenetic-mark-on-your-genes.

8. Farai Gundan, "Dr. Myles Munroe: On Leadership, Vision, Purpose and Maximizing Your Potential," *Forbes*, November 10, 2014, https://www.forbes.com/sites/faraigundan/2014/11/10/dr-myles-munroe-on-leadership-vision-purpose-and-maximizing-your-potential/#79ce9e913180.

CHAPTER 4
THE TOTAL COMPOSITION OF YOU

1. *Blue Letter Bible*, s.v. "pele'," accessed September 28, 2017, https://www.blueletterbible.org/lang/lexicon/lexicon.cfm?Strongs=H6382&t=KJV.

2. Derek Prince, "Spirit, Soul and Body" (letter), Derek Prince Ministries–US, accessed September 28, 2017, http://derekprince.org/Groups/1000065927/DPM_USA/Resources/Teaching_Articles/Teaching_Articles.aspx.

3. *Blue Letter Bible*, s.v. "*psychē*," accessed September 28, 2017, https://www.blueletterbible.org/lang/lexicon/lexicon.cfm?Strongs=G5590&t=KJV.

CHAPTER 5
TAMING THE SOUL

1. Shanelle Mullin, "The Advanced Guide to Emotional Persuasion," blog, August 11, 2017, accessed October 4, 2017, https://conversionxl.com/blog/emotional-persuasion-guide/.

2. Antonio Damasio, *Descartes' Error: Emotion, Reason, and the Human Brain* (New York: Penguin Books, 2005).

3. Frank Santora, *Turn It Around: A Different Direction for Your Life* (New York: Simon & Schuster, 2010), 165, https://books .google.com/books?id=UOKiCC6nCtQC&pg.

Chapter 6
Who Is Driving?

1. Tony Robbins, *Awaken the Giant Within* (New York: Simon & Schuster, 2007).
2. "Self-Help," *Wikipedia,* updated July 13, 2017, https://en .wikipedia.org/wiki/Self-help.
3. Frank Santora, in communication with the author.
4. Caroline Leaf, in communication with the author.

Chapter 7
The Body

1. M. Scott Peck, *The Road Less Traveled* (New York: Simon & Schuster, 2002), 64, https://books.google.com/books?id =KNyvQxE466kC&q.
2. Derek Grier, in communication with the author.
3. Joseph Clarino, in communication with the author.
4. "How Wounds Heal," *Medline Plus*, accessed October 4, 2017, https://medlineplus.gov/ency/patientinstructions/000741.htm.
5. Brett A. Morgan, "Inflammation: The Root of Illness and the Basis for Healing," *True Health*, accessed October 4, 2017, http://www.truehealthwv.com/nutrition-wellness/inflammation -information/.
6. Amanda MacMillan, "13 Ways Inflammation Can Affect Your Health," Health.com, March 4, 2015, accessed October 4, 2017, http://www.health.com/health/gallery/0,,20898778,00.html#too -much-of-a-good-thing--0.
7. MacMillan, "13 Ways Inflammation Can Affect Your Health."

8. Joseph Mercola, "7 Worst Ingredients in Food," Mercola.com, December 30, 2013, accessed October 4, 2017, https://articles .mercola.com/sites/articles/archive/2013/12/30/worst-food -ingredients.aspx; Tom Malterre, "Processed Foods: How Do They Affect Your Body?," *Whole Life Nutrition*, accessed October 4, 2017, https://wholelifenutrition.net/articles/gluten -free/processed-foods-how-do-they-affect-your-body.

9. M. K. Heliovaara, A. M. Teppo, S. L. Karonen, and P. Ebeling, "Inflammation Affects Lipid Metabolism During Recovery From Hyperinsulinaemia," *European Journal of Clinical Investigation* 36, no. 12 (December 2006): 860–865, abstract viewed October 4, 2017, at http://onlinelibrary.wiley.com/doi/10.1111 /j.1365-2362.2006.01730.x/abstract.

10. "Americans Get Less Sleep Than 20 Years Ago," CBSNews.com, February 28, 2008, accessed October 4, 2017, https://www .cbsnews.com/news/americans-get-less-sleep-than-20-years-ago/; Malcolm von Schantz, "Why Aren't We Getting Enough Sleep, and Why Does It Matter?," *British Counsel*, May 21, 2015, accessed October 4, 2017, https://www.britishcouncil.org/voices -magazine/why-arent-we-getting-enough-sleep-and-why-does-it -matter.

11. Denise Mann, "Sleep and Weight Gain," *WebMD*, reviewed April 30, 2013, accessed October 4, 2017, https://www.webmd .com/sleep-disorders/features/lack-of-sleep-weight-gain#1.

12. *Oxford English Dictionary*, s.v. "cognition," accessed September 30, 2017, https://en.oxforddictionaries.com/definition/cognition.

13. Camille Peri, "What Lack of Sleep Does to Your Mind," *WebMD*, reviewed April 30, 2013, accessed October 4, 2017, https://www.webmd.com/sleep-disorders/features/emotions -cognitive#1.

14. "Sleep and Disease Risk," *Healthy Sleep*, reviewed December 18, 2007, accessed October 5, 2017, http://healthysleep.med.harvard .edu/healthy/matters/consequences/sleep-and-disease-risk.

15. Paula Alhola and Paivi Polo-Kantola, "Sleep Deprivation: Impact on Cognitive Performance," *Neuropsychiatric Disease and Treatment* 3, no. 5 (October 2007): 553–567, abstract viewed October 5, 2017, https://www.ncbi.nlm.nih.gov/pmc /articles/PMC2656292/.

16. "Body Water," *Wikipedia*, last updated July 22, 2017, https:// en.wikipedia.org/wiki/Body_water.

17. "Functions of Water in the Body," *Mayo Clinic*, accessed October 5, 2017, http://www.mayoclinic.org/healthy-lifestyle /nutrition-and-healthy-eating/multimedia/functions-of-water -in-the-body/img-20005799.

18. "Prevent Diabetes Problems: Keep Your Kidneys Healthy," *National Institute of Diabetes and Digestive and Kidney Diseases*, accessed October 5, 2017, https://www.alohacare.org /userfiles/file/PDF/QUEST/Member/Health%20and%20 Wellness/5%20Keep%20Your%20Kidneys%20Healthy_2015.pdf.

19. Barry M. Popkin, Kristen E. D'Anci, and Irwin H. Rosenberg, "Water, Hydration and Health," *Nutrition Reviews* 68, no. 8 (August 1, 2010): 439–458, accessed October 5, 2017, https://academic.oup.com/nutritionreviews/article-lookup/doi/10.1111 /j.1753-4887.2010.00304.x.

20. K. C. Craichy, in communication with the author.

21. "The Four Ways We Kill Ourselves," *Living to 150* (blog), accessed September 30, 2017, http://livingto150.com/the-four -ways-we-kill-ourselves/.

22. "The Four Ways We Kill Ourselves," *Living to 150*.

23. "The Four Ways We Kill Ourselves," *Living to 150*.

24. Sergei I. Grivennikov, Florian R. Greten, and Michael Karin, "Immunity, Inflammation, and Cancer," *Cell* 140, no. 6 (March 19, 2010): 883–899, http://dx.doi.org/10.1016/j.cell.2010.01.025; Zoya Tahergorabi and Majid Khazaei, "The Relationship Between Inflammatory Markers, Angiogenesis, and Obesity," *ARYA Atherosclerosis* 9, no. 4 (June 2013): 247–253, https:// www.ncbi

.nlm.nih.gov/pmc/articles/PMC3746949/; Adriana Martorana, Matteo Bulati, Silvio Buffa, Mariavaleria Pellicanò, Calogero Caruso, Giuseppina Candore, and Giuseppina Colonna-Romano, "Immunosenescence, Inflammation and Alzheimer's Disease," *Longev Healthspan* 1 (2012): 8, doi: 10.1186/2046-2395-1-8.

25. "Glycation," *Wikipedia,* last updated August 10, 2017, https://en.wikipedia.org/wiki/Glycation.

26. "The Four Ways We Kill Ourselves," *Living to 150.*

27. Jeanine Barone, "The ABCs of AGEs (Advanced Glycation End-Products)," *Remedy Health Media, LLC*, February 28, 2017, http://www.berkeleywellness.com/healthy-eating/food-safety/article/abcs-ages-advanced-glycation-end-products.

28. "The Four Ways We Kill Ourselves," *Living to 150.*

29. Charbel Abi Khalil, "The Emerging Role of Epigenetics in Cardiovascular Disease," *Therapeutic Advances in Chronicic Disease* 5, no. 4 (July 2014): 178–187, doi: 10.1177/2040622314529325.

30. K. C. Craichy, in communication with the author.

31. James Hamblin, "1922: Strength and Vigor Depend on What You Eat," *The Atlantic*, April 1, 2014, https://www.theatlantic.com/health/archive/2014/04/1922-strength-and-vigor-depend-on-what-you-eat/284604/.

Chapter 8
Healing From the Inside

1. Kris Gunnars, "Does All Disease Really Begin in the Gut? The Surprising Truth," *HealthLine*, March 15, 2015, accessed October 10, 2017, https://www.healthline.com/nutrition/does-all-disease-begin-in-the-gut.

2. Morgan Chilson, "Symptoms of Leaky Gut Syndrome," *Newsmax Media Inc.*, September 8, 2015, http://www.newsmax

.com/FastFeatures/symptoms-leaky-gut-syndrome/2015/09/08
/id/678602/.

3. Elizabeth Doughman, "Mouse Study Links 'Leaky Gut' to
Chronic Inflammation," *ALN Magazine*, May 2, 2017, accessed
October 5, 2017, https://www.alnmag.com/news/2017/05/mouse
-study-links-leaky-gut-chronic-inflammation.

4. Russell Schierling, "Inflammation, Pain, Gluten, and the
Leakies," October 17, 2016, accessed October 5, 2017, http://
www.doctorschierling.com/blog/why-the-leakies-may-be
-decimating-your-health-and-what-you-can-do-about-it.

5. Schierling, "Inflammation, Pain, Gluten, and the Leakies."

6. Josh Axe, "5 Signs You Are Suffering From Candida
Overgrowth—and What You Can Do About It," *U.S. News and
World Report*, December 23, 2015, accessed October 5, 2017,
https://health.usnews.com/health-news/blogs/eat-run/articles
/2015-12-23/5-signs-youre-suffering-from-candida-overgrowth
-and-what-you-can-do-about-it.

7. Caroline Leaf, "Gut-Brain Connection," *Dr. Leaf's Blog*,
November 23, 2016, http://drleaf.com/blog/gut-brain
-connection/.

8. Leaf, "Gut-Brain Connection."

9. "Damon Davis Interviews Dr. Joel Wallach on 1onOne,"
TheWallachRevolution.com, accessed October 16, 2017, http://
thewallachrevolution.com/dr-wallach-damon-davis/; "Damon
Davis Interview With Dr. Joel Wallach Part 3," TheWallach
Revolution.com, accessed October 16, 2017, http://thewallach
revolution.com/damon-davis-interview-with-dr-joel-wallach
-part-3/.

10. "Damon Davis Interview With Dr. Joel Wallach Part 1,"
TheWallachRevolution.com, accessed October 16, 2017, http://
thewallachrevolution.com/damon-davis-interview-with-dr-joel
-wallach-pg-1/.

11. "Damon Davis Interview With Dr. Joel Wallach Part 1."

12. "Damon Davis Interview With Dr. Joel Wallach Part 2," TheWallachRevolution.com, accessed October 16, 2017, http://thewallachrevolution.com/damon-davis-interview-with-dr-joel-wallach-part-2/.

13. "Damon Davis Interview With Dr. Joel Wallach Part 2."

14. "Damon Davis Interview With Dr. Joel Wallach Part 2."

15. Joseph Christiano, "About Us," *Body Redesigning,* accessed October 9, 2017, http://www.bodyredesigning.net/about.asp.

16. Joseph Christiano, in communication with the author.

17. Christiano, in communication with the author.

18. Christiano, in communication with the author.

19. Christiano, in communication with the author.

20. Christiano, in communication with the author.

21. Joseph Christiano, *Bloodtypes, Bodytypes and You* (Lake Mary, FL: Siloam, 2004), 16, https://books.google.com/books?id=l8eGIZJpzTcC&.

22. Joseph Christiano, in communication with the author.

23. Creflo A. Dollar, *8 Steps to Create the Life You Want: The Anatomy of a Successful Life* (New York: FaithWords, 2008), 88–89, https://books.google.com/books?id=wqyvCABHyfsC&vq.

CHAPTER 9
DREAMING REAL DREAMS

1. Plato, quoted at *Quotes Area*, May 31, 2017, accessed October 9, 2017, http://www.quotesarea.com/music-and-rhythm-find/.

2. "Martin Luther's View on Music," *Grunewald,* accessed October 9, 2017, http://www.rjgrune.com/blog/martin-luthers-view-on-music.

3. Steve Eighinger, "Renowned Pianist to Play at Quincy Church," *Herald-Whig,* June 2, 2010, accessed October 9, 2017, http://www.whig.com/article/20080827/ARTICLE/308279985#.

4. Madeleine L'Engle, *Walking on Water: Reflections on Faith and Art* (New York: Crown Publishing Group, 2016), 8.

CHAPTER 10
THE JOURNEY

1. *Blue Letter Bible*, s.v. "*erchomai*," accessed October 2, 2017, https://www.blueletterbible.org/lang/lexicon/lexicon.cfm?Strongs=G2064&t=KJV.
2. *Blue Letter Bible*, s.v. "*zōē*," accessed October 2, 2017, https://www.blueletterbible.org/lang/lexicon/lexicon.cfm?Strongs=G2222&t=KJV.
3. "Vision," *Derek Grier Ministries*, accessed October 2, 2017, http://www.derekgrier.com/vision/.

CHAPTER 11
TWENTY-ONE DAYS TO DISCOVER THAT GOD CURES

1. "Weight Management," *Boston Medical Center*, accessed October 2, 2017, https://www.bmc.org/nutrition-and-weight-management/weight-management.
2. "Weight Management," *Boston Medical Center*.
3. Gina Shaw, "Could Losing Weight Ease Your Arthritis Pain?," *WebMD*, accessed October 2, 2017, https://www.webmd.com/osteoarthritis/features/lose-weight#1; Amy Gorin, "7 Reasons to Lose 5 Percent of Your Body Weight," Everyday Health Media, LLC, accessed October 2, 2017, https://www.everydayhealth.com/news/reasons-lose-5-percent-body-weight/.
4. Maxwell Maltz, *Psycho-Cybernetics* (New York: Simon & Schuster, 1989), xiii–xiv, https://books.google.com/books?id=J8dqtO6XqPMC&q.

5. Jason Selk, "Habit Formation: The 21-Day Myth," *Forbes*, April 15, 2013, https://www.forbes.com/sites/jasonselk/2013/04/15/habit-formation-the-21-day-myth/#58e55e07debc.

6. "WHO Report Says Eating Processed Meat Is Carcinogenic: Understanding the Findings," *Harvard School of Public Health*, accessed October 5, 2017, https://www.hsph.harvard.edu/nutritionsource/2015/11/03/report-says-eating-processed-meat-is-carcinogenic-understanding-the-findings/.

7. "WHO Report Says Eating Processed Meat Is Carcinogenic: Understanding the Findings," *Harvard School of Public Health*.

8. Maria Godoy, "Sugar Shocked? The Rest of Food Industry Pays for Lots of Research, Too," *National Public Radio*, September 14, 2016, accessed October 5, 2017, http://www.npr.org/sections/thesalt/2016/09/14/493957290/not-just-sugar-food-industry-s-influence-on-health-research.

9. "Meat Contamination," *PETA*, accessed October 5, 2017, https://www.peta.org/living/food/meat-contamination/.

10. Sylvain Charlebois, "Brazil and the Mother of All Food Fraud Cases," *Troy Media*, March 23, 2017, accessed October 5, 2017, http://www.ellinghuysen.com/news/articles/199100.shtml.

11. "How Much Dairy Does the Average American Consume in a Year?," *Washington State Journal*, June 23, 2017, accessed October 5, 2017, http://host.madison.com/wsj/business/how-much-dairy-does-the-average-american-consume-in-a/article_5f1e4abf-4442-548e-991d-f93e8afae95a.html.

12. Sandi Busch, "Recommended Daily Servings for Each of the Food Groups," LiveStrong.com, updated October 3, 2017, accessed October 2017, http://www.livestrong.com/article/361586-how-big-is-a-serving-size/.

13. Markham Heid, "Experts Say Lobbying Skewed the U.S. Dietary Guidelines," *TIME Health*, January 8, 2016, accessed October 5, 2017, http://time.com/4130043/lobbying-politics-dietary-guidelines/.

14. Paige Fowler, "Read This Before You Give Up Dairy," *Rodale Organic Life*, October 13, 2005, accessed October 5, 2017, https://www.rodalesorganiclife.com/food/read-this-before-you-give-up-dairy.

15. "Lactose Intolerance," *U.S. National Library of Medicine*, accessed October 5, 2017, https://ghr.nlm.nih.gov/condition/lactose-intolerance#definition.

16. "7 Symptoms of Lactose Intolerance and Diet to Treat It," DrAxe.com, accessed October 5, 2017, https://draxe.com/symptoms-of-lactose-intolerance/.

CONNECT WITH US!

(Spiritual Growth)

f Facebook.com/CharismaHouse

y @CharismaHouse

O Instagram.com/CharismaHouse

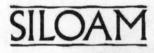

(Health)

P Pinterest.com/CharismaHouse

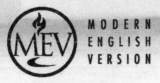

(Bible)

www.mevbible.com

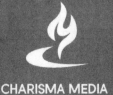